WITHDRAWN
WRIGHT STATE UNIVERSITY LIBRARIES

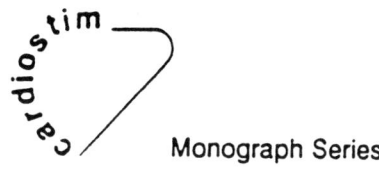

Monograph Series

Noninvasive Transcutaneous Cardiac Pacing

Edited by:

Pierre J. Birkui, MD, FICA
Research Associate INSERM
Clinique Cardiologique
Hopital Lariboisiere
Paris, France

Jacques A. Trigano, MD
Department of Cardiac Pacing
Centre Hospitalier Universitaire
C.H.U. Marseille Nord
Marseille, France

Paul M. Zoll, MD
Clinical Professor of Medicine Emeritus
Harvard Medical School
Beth Israel Hospital
Department of Medicine
Boston, Massachusetts

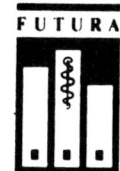

Futura Publishing
Company, Inc.
Mount Kisco, NY

Library of Congress Cataloging-in-Publication Data

Noninvasive transcutaneous cardiac pacing / edited by Pierre J. Birkui, Jacques A. Trigano, Paul M. Zoll.
    p.   cm. — (Cardiostim monograph series)
  Includes index.
  1. Cardiac pacing. I. Birkui, Pierre J. II. Trigano, Jacques A. III. Zoll, Paul M. IV. Series.
  [DNLM: 1. Cardiac Pacing, Artificial—methods.
2. Electrophysiology. WG 168 N813]
RC684.P3N66 1993
617.4'120645—dc20
DNLM/DLC
for Library of Congress   92-22267
                                                                                   CIP

Copyright 1993
Futura Publishing Company, Inc.

Published by
Futura Publishing Company, Inc.
2 Bedford Ridge Road
Mount Kisco, New York 10549

L.C. No.: 92-22267
ISBN No.: 0-87993-5367

Every effort has been made to ensure that the information in this book is as up to date and accurate as possible at the time of publication. However, due to the constant developments in medicine, neither the author, nor the editor, nor the publisher can accept any legal or any other responsibility for any errors or omissions that may occur.

All rights reserved.
No part of this book may be translated or reproduced in any form without written permission of the publisher.

Printed in the United States of America on acid-free paper.

Contributors

Glenn E. Aldinger, MD, FACEP Assistant Clinical Professor of Surgery, Loyola University Stritch School of Medicine, Maywood, Illinois, Chairman, Department of Emergency Medicine, Saint Francis Hospital of Evanston, Evanston, Illinois

Giuliano Altamura, MD Director of Pacing and Clinical Electrophysiology Laboratory, Division of Cardiology, San Filippo Neri Hospital, Rome, Italy

Marie J. Beland, MDCM, FRCP (C) Assistant Professor of Pediatrics, McGill University; Associate Director, Division of Cardiology, The Montreal Children's Hospital, Montreal, Canada

Leopoldo Bianconi, MD Vice Director, Cardiology Clinic, Division of Cardiology, San Filippo Neri Hospital, Rome, Italy

Pierre J. Birkui, MD, FICA Research Associate INSERM, Clinique Cardiologique, Hopital Lariboisiere, Paris, France

William C. Dalsey, MD, MBA, FACEP Associate Professor of Medicine, Temple University; Chairman, Department of Emergency Medicine, Albert Einstein Medical Center, Philadelphia, Pennsylvania

Thomas F. Deering, MD Director, Cardiac Electrophysiology Laboratory, Piedmont Hospital; Assistant Clinical Professor, Georgia Baptist Medical Center, Atlanta, Georgia

Jean Degonde, PhD Electronic Engineer, Engineer Associate INSERM, Hopital Lariboisiere Paris, France

Arthur R. Easley Jr, MD Assistant professor of Medicine, Division of Cardiology, University of Nebraska Medical Center, Omaha, Nebraska

N.A. Mark Estes III, MD Professor of Medicine-Tufts University School of Medicine; Director-Cardiac Electrophysiology and Pacemaker Laboratory, New England Medical Center Hospitals, Boston, Massachusetts

Jerzy Galecka, Dipl. Eng. Electronic Engineer, Medical Electronics E.A.M. Center OBREAM, Zabrze, Poland

Jerris R. Hedges, MD, MS, FACEP Associate Professor of Emergency Medicine, Director of Research Programs, Oregon Health Sciences University, Division of Emergency Medicine, Portland, Oregon

Krzysztof Jarczok, MD The Silesian Medical Academy, The First Department of Internal Disease, Katowice, Poland

Carolyn J. Kenyon, MD Department of Medicine, Section of Emergency Medicine, Charity Hospital of New Orleans, New Orleans, Louisiana

Francesco Lo Bianco, MD Staff Cardiologist, Pacing and Electrophysiology Laboratory, Division of Cardiology, San Filippo Neri Hospital, Rome, Italy

Jerry C. Luck, MD Associate Professor of Medicine, Division of Cardiology, The Milton S. Hershey Medical Center, The Pennsylvania State University, Hershey, Pennsylvania

Jan Kyst Madsen, MD, DMSc Lecturer in Medicine, Senior Registrar, Department of Medicine B, Rigshospitalet, University of Copenhagen, Copenhagen, Denmark

Antonis S. Manolis, MD Assistant Professor of Medicine-Tufts University School of Medicine, Associate Director-Cardiac Electrophysiology and Pacemaker Laboratory, New England Medical Center Hospitals, Boston, Massachusetts

Michael L. Markel, MD Division of Cardiology, The Milton S. Hershey Medical Center, The Pennsylvania State University, Hershey, Pennsylvania

Fryderyk Prochaczek, MD The Silesian Medical Academy, The First Department of Internal Disease, Katowice, Poland

Deeb Salem, MD Professor of Medicine, Tufts University School of Medicine; Chief, Division of Cardiology, New England Medical Center Hospitals, Boston, Massachusetts

Massimo Santini, MD, FACC Director, Division of Cardiology, San Filippo Neri Hospital, Rome, Italy

Peter Schulman, MD, FACC   Associate Professor of Medicine, The University of Connecticut Health Center, Farmington, Connecticut

Robert A. Stratbucker, MD, PhD   Associate Professor of Radiology, University of Nebraska Medical Center, Omaha, Nebraska

Salvatore Toscano, MD   Vice Director, Pacing and Clinical Electrophysiology Laboratory, Division of Cardiology, San Filippo Neri Hospital, Rome, Italy

Jacques A. Trigano, MD   Department of Cardiac Pacing, Centre Hospitalier Universitaire, C.H.U. Marseille Nord, Marseille, France

Fernand Vandamme, PhD   Professor of Applied Epistemology, The Baggage Institute for Knowledge and Information Technology (BIKIT), Lab-Applied Epistemology, University of Ghent, Ghent, Belgium

Michel Verheyen, MA   Researcher, The Baggage Institute for Knowledge and Information Technology (BIKIT), Lab Applied Epistemology, University of Ghent, Ghent, Belgium

John R. Windle, MD   Associate Chief of Cardiology, Associate Professor of Medicine, Division of Cardiology, University of Nebraska Medical Center, Omaha, Nebraska

Paul M. Zoll, MD   Clinical Professor of Medicine, Emeritus, Harvard Medical School, Beth Israel Hospital, Department of Medicine, Boston, Massachusetts

Ross H. Zoll, MD, PhD   Anesthesiologist, Providence Anesthesia Associates, Holyoke, Massachusetts

Introduction

For the past 40 years, it has been known that electric stimulation can act as a substitute for the physiologic heart stimulus when the latter is failing. This concept of external cardiac pacing in humans was first supplemented by Zoll and then by Coraboeuf and Zacouto in 1952–1953.

During the first clinical attempts at pacing, stimulation was transmitted to the myocardium via a transcutaneous route with safety-pin electrodes under the skin on both sides of the anterior precordial chest. This method was capable of inducing systolic myocardial contractions, but it also induced vigorous contractions of the chest, arms, or abdominal muscles, which caused intolerable pain.

In October, 1960 at the Lariboisiére Hospital in Paris, we were given the chance to use a painless method that had been introduced by Dr. Seymour Furman some weeks previously. A 55-year-old woman presented with an atrioventricular block. Suddenly, the Stokes-Adams attacks became fulgurant and electrosystolic transcutaneous pacing was impossible. What was to be done? With a catheter from the hemodynamic laboratory, we installed an electric lead. For this purpose, a metallic guide was introduced slightly beyond the distal part of the catheter. The proximal part of the catheter was connected to the negative pole of a pulse generator set at 8 volts. It was not without apprehension that I decided to insert this improvised tool into a vein of the arm and push it up to the right ventricle. I had no idea what would happen or how the myocardium would respond to receiving this direct electrostimulus on the endocardium. We had only the single precedent described by Furman and coworkers as a guide for the procedure. Despite our fears, everything went smoothly and electrosystolic pacing was maintained for several days without resultant pain. In the ensuing time period our rudimentary equipment was improved, and we had many opportunities to use it for temporary stimulation.

In following years, the first implanted devices became available. However, the large size of these devices and the discomfort their implantation caused were major disadvantages. In addition, the leads, which often broke, were positioned on the epicardium, which required thoracotomy, and there were breakdowns of the primary generators. Moreover, this was an unreliable mode of stimulation because it paced the heart regardless of its underlying rhythm.

During the past 30 years, improvements in pacing devices culminated in the development of "intelligent" miniaturized pacemakers equipped with external controls. During that same time period, however, there was no progress made by technicians and cardiologists towards adapting a technique capable of inducing quick and painless temporary electrosystolic pacing. Such a technique would be very useful in cases where we have reason to predict that an AV block may be temporary or when we are unable to install an efficient intracavitary lead. Until recently, the archaic method of pacing was still used in such cases.

Fortunately, a persistent research worker, Dr. P.M. Zoll, became the first to develop an effective method of electrosystolic transcutaneous pacing that was easy to use, quickly operational, and painless. This breakthrough was followed by numerous studies and publications worldwide, including those of Birkui, Trigano, and Degonde in France.

The purpose of this monograph is to present the results of these studies and disseminate this important information that will be valuable to physicians and patients alike.

Pr. Yves Bouvrain

Contents

Contributors	....	iii
Introduction	Pr. Yves Bouvrain	vii

I. BASICS

Chapter 1. Cardiac Activation by Noninvasive Cardiac Pacing
Giuliano Altamura, MD, Salvatore Toscano, MD, Leopoldo Bianconi, MD, Francesco Lo Bianco, MD, Massimo Santini, MD, FACC 3

Chapter 2. Tolerance and Pacing Threshold with Noninvasive Transcutaneous Cardiac Pacing
Pierre J. Birkui, MD, FICA, Jacques A. Trigano, MD, Jean Degonde, PhD 13

II. BIOLOGICAL ASPECTS

Chapter 3. Myocardial Enzyme Monitoring Pacing
Jan Kyst Madsen, MD, DMSc 33

III. HEMODYNAMIC STUDIES

Chapter 4. The Hemodynamics of External Cardiac Pacing
Peter Schulman, MD, FACC 41

IV. EMERGENCY MANAGEMENT

Chapter 5. Transcutaneous Cardiac Pacing in Cardiac Arrest
William C. Dalsey, MD, FACEP 49

Chapter 6. Emergency Prehospital Transcutaneous Cardiac Pacing
Jerris R. Hedges, MD, MS, FACEP 61

Chapter 7. Prehospital Prospective Controlled
Transcutaneous Cardiac Pacing:
24-Month Clinical Trial
Carolyn J. Kenyon, MD,
Glenn E. Aldinger, MD, FACEP 75

V. APPLICATION IN CHILDREN

Chapter 8. Noninvasive Transcutaneous Cardiac
Pacing in Children
Marie J. Beland, MDCM, FRCP (C) 91

VI. PROGRESS IN CLINICAL ELECTROPHYSIOLOGY

Chapter 9. Noninvasive Cardiac Stimulation,
Fibrillation, and Defibrillation
Paul M. Zoll, MD,
Ross H. Zoll, MD, PhD 101

Chapter 10. Noninvasive Transcutaneous Cardiac
Pacing for Termination of Ventricular
and Supraventricular Tachycardias
Giuliano Altamura, MD,
Leopoldo Bianconi, MD,
Salvatore Toscano, MD,
Francesco Lo Bianco, MD,
Massimo Santini, MD 107

Chapter 11. Noninvasive Cardiac Pacing for Ventricular
Tachycardia: Feasibility of
Electrophysiological Testing
Jerry C. Luck, MD,
Michael L. Markel, MD 119

Chapter 12. Noninvasive Transcutaneous Cardiac
Pacing for Termination of Sustained
Supraventricular and Ventricular
Tachycardias
N.A. Mark Estes III, MD,
Thomas F. Deering, MD,
Antonis S. Manolis, MD,
Deeb Salem, MD,
Paul M. Zoll, MD 131

VII. ECHOCARDIOGRAPHIC ASPECT

Chapter 13. Echocardiographic Evaluation of Left Ventricular Function During Noninvasive Transcutaneous Cardiac Pacing
Jan Kyst Madsen, MD, DMSc 149

VIII. NEW APPLICATIONS

Chapter 14. New Clinical Applications of Noninvasive Transcutaneous Cardiac Pacing
Fryderyk Prochaczek, MD, Jerzy Galecka, Dipl. Eng., Krzysztof Jarczok, MD 161

Chapter 15. A Multipurpose Self-Adhesive Patch Electrode Capable of External Pacing, Cardioversion/Defibrillation, and 12-Lead Electrocardiogram
John R. Windle, MD, Arthur R. Easley, Jr, MD, Robert A. Stratbucker, PhD, MD 179

Chapter 16. Knowledge Systems, Expert Systems, Medicine, and Noninvasive Transcutaneous Cardiac Pacing
Fernand Vandamme, PhD, Michel Verheyen, MA 193

Chapter 17. Noninvasive Transcutaneous Cardiac Pacing: Current Devices and Related Products
Jacques A. Trigano, MD, Pierre J. Birkui, MD, FICA 205

Index 219

I

Basics

Chapter 1

Cardiac Activation by Noninvasive Cardiac Pacing

Giuliano Altamura, MD, Salvatore Toscano, MD, Leopoldo Bianconi, MD, Francesco Lo Bianco, MD, Massimo Santini, MD

In the early 1980s, significant technological advances concerning the electrode's surface and electrical pulses characteristics have improved the reliability and the tolerability of noninvasive transcutaneous cardiac pacing (NTCP).[1]

Several studies compared NTCP with endocavitary stimulation. The hemodynamic effects of ventricular stimulation obtained by the two techniques were reported to be comparable.[2,3] Left ventricular pressure measurements were found to be similar, while cardiac output increased significantly during NTCP, suggesting a favorable hemodynamic effect of muscular chest wall stimulation.[4]

By echocardiographic methods, external cardiac pacing was seen to produce a simultaneous contraction of the two ventricles.[5] This is in contradistinction to right ventricle endocavitary stimulation, where left ventricular activation delay produces a typical abnormal movement of interventricular septum, analogous to that observed in left bundle branch block.

Actually, during external pacing, a four chamber biatrial and biventricular activation has been hypothesized.[6,7] So far, this phenomenon has been verified, by endocavitary recording, only in

From *Noninvasive Transcutaneous Cardiac Pacing* edited by Pierre Birkui, M.D., Jacques Trigano, M.D., and Paul Zoll, M.D., © 1993, Futura Publishing Company, Inc., Mount Kisco, NY.

animal models.[8] However, in subsequent human studies, performed by transesophageal or endocavitary recording, NTCP was not found to be able to directly capture the atria.[9-11] Moreover, atrioventricular dissociation or ventriculoatrial retroconduction was reported by means of endocavitary or transesophageal recording[12-14] and echocardiographic methods.[5] Both findings exclude atrial capture by external pacing.

These contrasting reports prompted us to examine again the issue of cardiac activation by NTCP, focusing on the timing of atrial and ventricular depolarization.

Materials and Methods

We studied nine patients (six males, three females), mean age 62 years (range:35 to 81), undergoing electrophysiological studies for different reasons (atrioventricular conduction or vulnerability evaluation). After obtaining the patient's consent, NTCP was performed in all of them and atrial and ventricular endocavitary recordings were obtained. The noninvasive pacing device we used was the Pace Aid® model 52 (Cardiac Resuscitator Corporation, Oregon, USA) that can perform a constant current stimulation at 9 programmable outputs (10, 20, 40, 50, 60, 70, 80, 100, and 150 mA) and 20 msec pulse width. The pace rates range from 50 to 160 ppm. During pacing, ECG recording of the cardiac electrical activity is made possible thanks to a "pulse blanking" circuit.[1]

The pregelled high impedance electrodes, with a stimulation surface area of about 50 cm^2, were placed anteriorly in electrocardiographic V3 position and posteriorly between left scapula and spine at the cardiac level. Endocavitary quadripolar leads used for recording were positioned in high right atrium and right ventricular apex.

All the patients were studied while in sinus rhythm and the possibility of atrial capture by endocavitary pacing was preventively demonstrated. NTCP, at a rate about of 30% above the spontaneous sinus rhythm, was performed starting with a current output of 40 mA. The current intensity was then increased until atrial capture was achieved or the maximum pacing energy was reached. At every stimulation energy, the pacing was applied for no more than 10 sec. Ventricular and atrial pacing threshold and atrial retrograde activation were evaluated.

After every externally delivered spike, there is a period of 40–60 msec, resulting from pulse width and postpolarization phenomena, during which intracavitary cardiac recording is hindered. Thus, the ventricular capture was inferred by disappearance, on the electrogram, of the spontaneous V waves and the presence of the T waves following the pacemaker spike. During ventricular pacing, atrial capture was deduced only when previously evident dissociated or retroconducted A waves constantly disappeared from intracavitary recording because they were hidden in the pacemaker artefacts (Fig. 1).

Every drug theoretically able to modify the stimulation threshold was withdrawn at least four half lives before the study. A premedication with intravenous diazepam was used to relieve the discomfort of high energy transcutaneous pacing and to obtain an artefact-free recording.

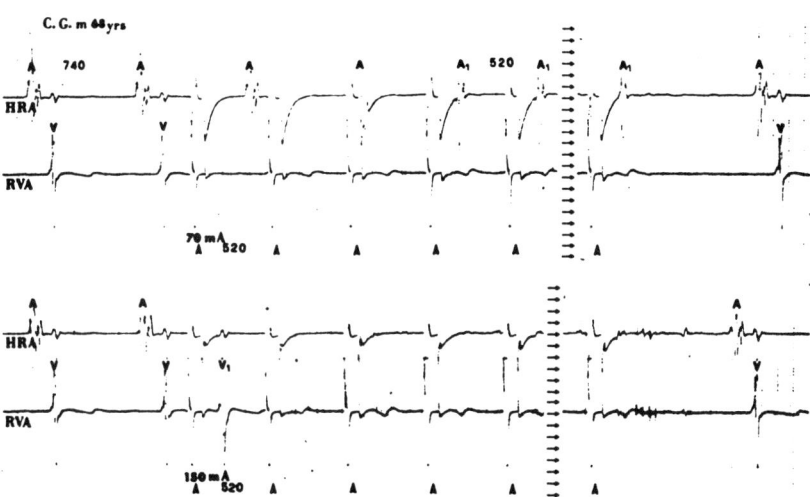

Figure 1. *Endocavitary recording (50 mm/sec) in high right atrium (HRA) and right ventricular apex (RVA) during sinus rhythm (period = 740 msec) and NTCP (period = 520 msec). Upper Strip: During NTCP (current output = 70 mA), all the stimuli, except the first one that falls in the ventricular refractory period, capture the ventricles (V waves are hindered into the pacing artefact and only repolarization is visible). Dissociated atrial activity (A-A = 740 msec) is present during the first three stimuli, then atrial retroactivation (A_1) appears. Lower strip: NTCP at 150 mA. The first stimulus falls in the ventricular refractory period. It captures only the atria and is followed by a conducted ventriculogram (V_1), the subsequent stimuli induce a simultaneous atrial and ventricular depolarization. Although neither A or V waves are visible, their presence inside the wide spike artefact can be inferred from the presence of T waves following the spike and from the absence of either dissociated or retroconducted A waves.*

Results

By means of NTCP, ventricular capture was obtained in all the nine patients with a mean current threshold of 74±14 mA, while simultaneous atrial and ventricular capture was observed in only four cases (44%), even at the maximum energy delivered (150 mA) (Table 1). The pulse strength necessary to capture the atria was 100 mA in one case and 150 mA in three cases (mean threshold: 138±25 mA). In one of these patients, intermittent 2:1 atrial capture was observed, at a pacing output of 150 mA (Fig. 2).

Retrograde atrial activation was present in five patients (56%).

At the highest energy stimulations employed, the majority of patients reported severe discomfort. No cutaneous damage at the electrode sites nor other untoward effects were observed.

Discussion

According to a previous study in dogs,[8] our results demonstrate that even in humans it is possible to obtain atrial capture by NTCP. In previous human studies,[5,9-14] atrial capture was never observed. This can be explained by the fact that in these studies, the pacing energies employed were lower, since the protocols used were designed to evaluate the ventricular activation. In fact, we used energies consider-

Table 1. Cardiac Activation by NTCP

Patient	Age (yrs)	Ventricular threshold (mA)	Atrial threshold (mA)	VA retro-conduction
1	65	80	—	yes
2	35	80	150	no
3	68	70	150	yes
4	76	70	—	no
5	54	50	100	yes
6	81	70	150*	yes
7	47	70	—	no
8	69	100	—	yes
9	63	80	—	no

*intermittent 2:1 atrial capture

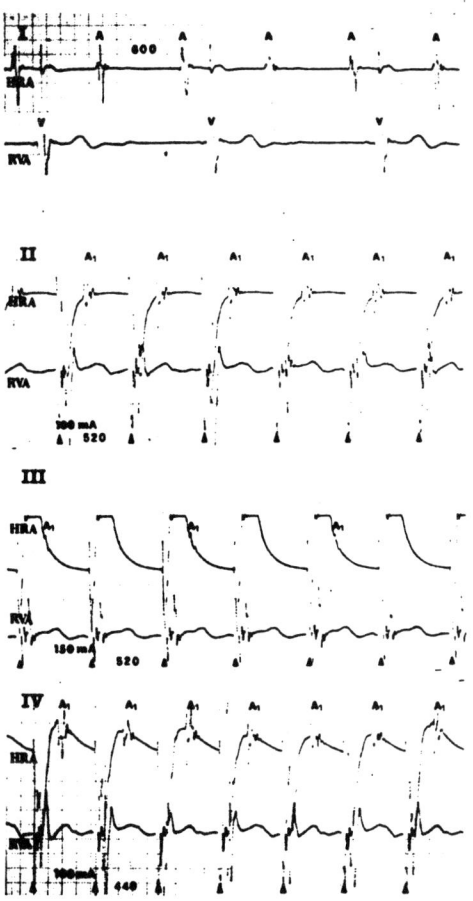

Figure 2. *Endocavitary recordings (50 mm/sec) in high right atrium (HRA) and right ventricular apex (RVA). Strip I: Sinus rhythm (A-A = 600 msec) with 2:1 atrioventricular block. Strip II: NTCP (stimulation period = 520 msec, current output = 100 mA): ventricular capture followed by constant atrial retroactivation (V-A_1 = 190 msec). Strip III: 150mA NTCP at the same period ventricular capture alternately followed by atrial retroactivation (V-A_1 = 190 msec). Strip IV: NTCP (period 440 msec, 100 mA): ventricular capture followed by constant atrial activation. In strip III, the alternate retroconduction and the absence of any A wave during a long A_1-A_1 interval (1040 msec) in a patient with normal sinus function (strip I) indicate intermittent atrial capture by NTCP. In fact, atrial retroconduction with 2:1 block can be excluded by the demonstration of constant retroconduction at higher stimulation rates and lower output current (strip IV).*

ably higher than those necessary for ventricular capture. In the only study[10] where high energy impulses (up to 140 mA) were employed, the failure to capture the atria could be due to differences in electrodes surface area, electrodes location, and pacing pulse width. For the purpose of our study, the stimulation device available to us has a limitation. It permits a wide choice of stimulation energies at lower current strength (10 mA steps until 80 mA), while at higher energy levels only two output currents are available (100 and 150 mA). This limited the possibility of precisely determining the atrial capture levels over 100 mA. Actually, in two patients in whom constant atrial capture was obtained with 150 mA, an atrial threshold slightly superior to 100 mA cannot be excluded. In the patient in which 2:1 atrial capture was obtained at the maximum pacing output, the threshold was obviously 150 mA.

The possibility of obtaining four chamber stimulation is not relevant for the main clinical indication of NTCP: the treatment of severe bradyarrhythmias. In this case, simultaneous atrial and ventricular capture could rather be disadvantageous. Indeed, an atrial contraction against closed atrioventricular valves can result in a negative hemodynamic effect, mainly by decreasing peripheral arterial resistance by a reflex mechanism.[15]

Moreover, the high current level necessary to obtain atrial capture and the consequent insufficient tolerance of the pacing by the patients render the method unsuitable for the electrophysiological evaluation of sinus function. Atrioventricular conduction is obviously not evaluable by NTCP because of the impossibility of obtaining atrial stimulation without ventricular capture due to the higher atrial than ventricular threshold.

However, the demonstration of the possibility of atrial capture in humans is important because it improves our knowledge of the effects of NTCP.

Moreover, this observation can offer a theoretical base for application of NTCP in the treatment of supraventricular reentrant tachycardias. In fact, high energy bursts, able to depolarize the four cardiac chambers, have more probability of penetrating the reentrant circuit than isolated atrial or ventricular stimulation.

Actually, in atrioventricular reentrant tachycardia, simultaneous atrial and ventricular capture is difficult or rather impossible to obtain because of the peculiar relationship between the ventricular and the subsequent atrial refractory periods. In fact, in this arrhythmia, the possibility of simultaneous four chamber stimulation by pacing is confined to the short period, not always present, between the end of atrial refractoriness and the beginning of the next ventricular depolarization.

In one of our patients, affected by a concealed bypass tract, we tested the NTCP during the electrophysiological study in order to interrupt the tachycardia (190 ppm) repeatedly induced by endocavitary programmed stimulation. The ventricular threshold was 70 mA and the atrial one 150 mA. NTCP, applied many times during different tachycardia episodes, with a current intensity of 150 mA at different rates (50, 80, and 150 ppm), repeatedly and very easily interrupted the tachycardia (Fig. 3) either by ventricular or atrial capture. We never observed simultaneous four chamber capture. It is worth noting that endocavitary underdrive ventricular pacing was never able to interrupt the tachycardia (Fig. 4). In this case, perhaps, the different pattern of ventricular activation could be the critical point accounting for the different ability of the two pacing modalities in interrupting the arrhythmia.

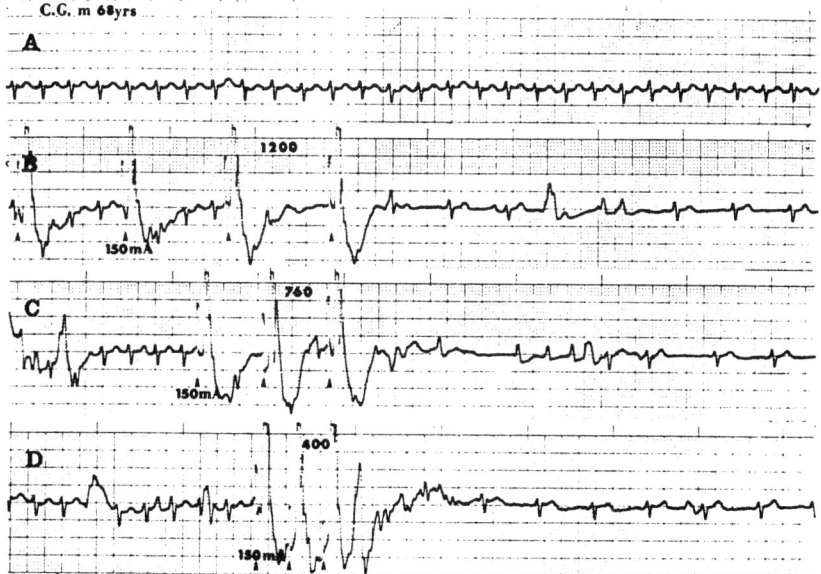

Figure 3. *A) Atrioventricular reentrant tachycardia (190 ppm) induced during electrophysiological study (recording obtained with Pace Aid model 52). Different tachycardia episodes terminated by NTCP, respectively at 50 (B), 80 (C), and 160 ppm (D).*

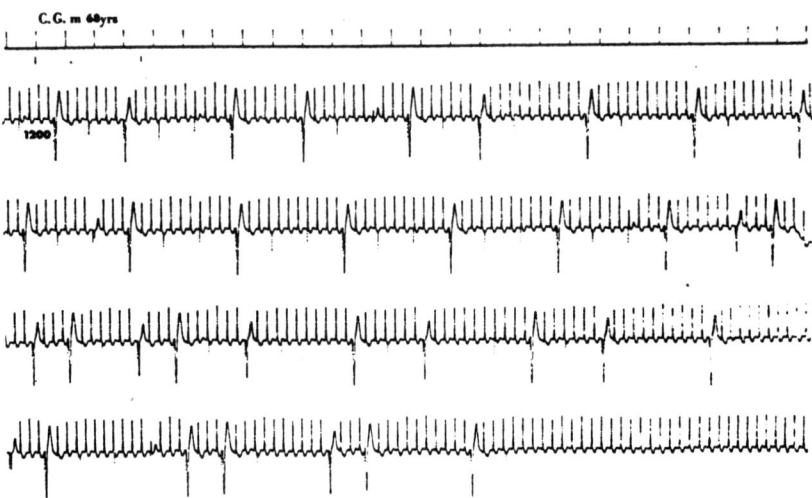

Figure 4. *Same patient as in Fig. 3. Continuous ECG strip (12.5 mm/sec) during tachycardia. Endocardial underdrive pacing applied for more than 120 sec at 50 ppm, while frequently capturing the ventricle, does not interrupt the tachycardia.*

Conclusion

Our data indicate that NTCP at medium current outputs induces only ventricular capture, followed by atrial depolarization when retroconduction is present. Higher energy stimulations, usually ill-tolerated by the patients, can produce simultaneous atrial and ventricular capture. The clinical utilization of this possibility is probably limited, but atrial capture could give to NTCP an additional chance for the interruption of supraventricular reentrant tachycardias.

References

1. Zoll PM: External noninvasive electric stimulation of the heart. Crit Care Med 9:393, 1981.
2. Niemann JT, Rosborugh JP, Garner D, et al.: External noninvasive cardiac pacing: A comparative hemodynamic study of two techniques with conventional endocardial pacing. PACE 7:230, 1984.
3. Syverud SA, Hedges GR, Dalsey WC, et al.: Hemodynamics of transcutaneous cardiac pacing. Am J Emerg Med 4:17, 1986.

4. Trigano JA, Remond JM, Mourot F, et al.: Left ventricular pressure during transcutaneous pacing (Abstr). PACE 11(Suppl):856, 1988.
5. Madsen JK, Pederson F, Grande P, et al.: Normal myocardial enzymes and normal echocardiographic findings during noninvasive transcutaneous pacing. PACE 11:1188, 1988.
6. Zipes DP: Electrical therapy of cardiac arrhythmias. N Engl J Med 309:1179, 1983.
7. Noe R, Cockrell W, Moses HW, et al.: Transcutaneous pacemaker use in a large hospital. PACE 9 (Part I):101, 1986.
8. Varghese PJ, Bren J, Ross A: Electrophysiology of external pacing: A comparative study with endocardial pacing (Abstr). Circulation 66(Suppl 2): 349, 1982.
9. Falk RH, Ngai STA, Kumaki DJ, et al.: Cardiac activation during external cardiac pacing. PACE 10 (Part I):503, 1987.
10. Luck JC, Grubb BP, Artman SE, et al.: Termination of sustained ventricular tachycardia by external noninvasive pacing. Am J Cardiol 61:574, 1988.
11. Klein LS, Miles WM, Heger JJ, et al.: Transcutaneous pacing: Patient tolerance, stength interval relations and feasibility for programmed electrical stimulation. Am J Cardiol 62:1126, 1988.
12. Luck JC, Davis D: Termination of sustained tachycardia by external noninvasive pacing. PACE 10:1125, 1987.
13. Markel ML, Grubb BP, Artman S, et al.: Effect of electrode location on ventricular activation and threshold during external pacing: Implication for programmed stimulation (Abstr). RBM 3:87, 1990.
14. Prochaczek F, Gadecka J, Machalski, et al.: Diagnostic transcutaneous cardiac pacing: Examination of the ventriculoatrial conduction (Abstr). PACE 11:856, 1988.
15. Alicandri C, Fouad RC, Tarazi L, et al.: Three cases of hypotension and syncope with ventricular pacing: Possible role of atrial reflexes. Am J Cardiol 42:137, 1978.

Chapter 2

Tolerance and Pacing Threshold with Noninvasive Transcutaneous Cardiac Pacing

Pierre J. Birkui, MD, FICA,
Jacques A. Trigano, MD, Jean Degonde, PhD

The substitution of an artificial stimulus with adequate parameters for the electrophysiological stimulus was already discussed more than a hundred years ago. Thus in 1872, Duchenne de Boulogne[1] wrote: "The rhythmic electrical stimulation over the precordium, around the apical myocardial zone, is one of the best ways to fight against cardiac arrest syncope." In 1889, Mac William[2] published an article on the electrical stimulation of the heart, differentiating between the cardiac arrest caused by asystole and that caused by ventricular fibrillation, and discussing the technique of what was called noninvasive transcutaneous cardiac pacing (NTCP). Much later, in 1952, this method was first implemented in the United States by PM Zoll,[3] using a ground electrode attached to the skin and a subcutaneous needle electrode over the precordial chest. The method was then used in France by Levy Solal, Donzelot, et al.[4,5]

During the years that followed, transvenous temporary pacing was described by Furman et al.,[6] and introduced and developed in France by Bouvrain et al.[7] As this technique requires time, experience in catheterization, and access to fluoroscopy, it cannot be used in an

---

From *Noninvasive Transcutaneous Cardiac Pacing* edited by Pierre Birkui, M.D., Jacques Trigano, M.D., and Paul Zoll, M.D., © 1993, Futura Publishing Company, Inc., Mount Kisco, NY.

emergency. In the same way as for ventricular tachycardia (VT) and fibrillation (VF) which both require cardioversion, bradyarrhythmia or asystole is the most common rhythm disturbance (30%-40% of cases) in which noninvasive cardiac pacing constitutes a prompt and very useful prehospital procedure prior to the initiation of support therapy in an intensive care unit or emergency department.

Articles on human and experimental NTCP applications often have an introduction recalling the first application in humans by PM Zoll.[3] After a gap of three decades, the history of this method resumed during the last decade (1982–92).

Why has this method, which has long been available as a first emergency therapy for bradyarrhythmia or asystole, not had the extraordinary development of endovenous pacing which was introduced later? At first, poor tolerance, muscle contractions, and skin burns were usual with NTCP because of electrode characteristics and high current density. The duration of the stimulus was equal to the myocardial chronaxia (about 3 msec in normal cardiac muscle).

The efficacy of NTCP is indisputable because many studies have demonstrated its hemodynamic benefit under various human, clinical, and experimental conditions. The indications and applications of NTCP have broadened since 1980, when it became more attractive,[8] and the former painful reactions were almost abolished by the use of new types of low ionic gel, longer impulses, larger electrode pads and a more effective contact between the skin and the electrode. Noninvasive external or transcutaneous cardiac pacing became one of the preferred methods of pacing the heart in emergency routine (Fig. 1). Nevertheless, discomfort may still occur in rare cases due to chest muscle and cutaneous nerve stimulation and might be increased by

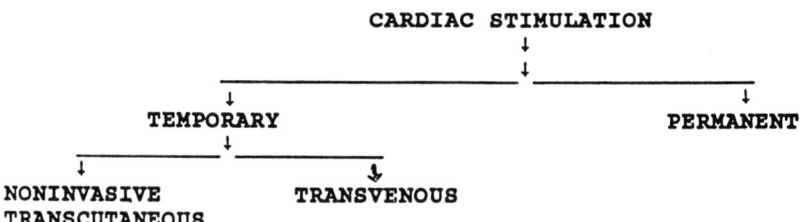

Figure 1. *Panel of cardiac stimulation, temporary or permanent, noninvasive or invasive, used in emergency situations, as therapy for conduction problems.*

current amplitude. Tolerance should be improved by the reduced ventricular pacing threshold. All that has been done to lower this threshold should lead to more widespread use of this emergency technique.

This study is a review of the correlations found between tolerance and pacing threshold on the one hand, and the effect of positioning and gel impedance electrodes on the other, in studies using large adhesive electrodes.

Tolerance

The discomfort caused by NTCP is due to skeletal muscle and cutaneous nerve chest stimulation with the increase of the current threshold. Various methods used to reduce this threshold have increased tolerance. One of them consisted of increasing the surface of the active anterior electrode. The most spectacular decrease in threshold (78%) was observed by Alferness et al.[9] with six pairs of electrodes in anterior and posterior positions around the canine chest which maintained the negative polarity in the anterior position. The threshold was around 115 mA with a single pair of anterior-posterior (AP) electrodes, 35 mA with three pairs, and 25 mA with six pairs. Each electrode had the same surface area, which was not, however, specified.

This substantial reduction in current density suggests that it would be appropriate to use several pairs of electrodes with a small surface area arranged on a large extensible chest belt so as to apply less current. This was already proposed in 1953 by Zacouto[10] for transcutaneous stimulation and also for external defibrillation. To reduce electrolysis, the delivery of alternate negative and positive impulses was also proposed.

Numerous studies of normal human volunteers as well as animal experiments failed to explore the possible correlation between tolerance and the amplitude of current density.

Using five transcutaneous pacing devices (Life Pak8, Physio Control; Pace Aid 53®, Cardiac Resuscitator Corp; Redipace, MDE; Transpace, MDI; and Zoll NTP) in ten healthy males, 25–39 years old, weighing 65 to 120 kg, Heller et al.[11] found that eight of the subjects displayed successful electrical capture with the Zoll NTP device at a mean threshold of 66.5 mA. Nevertheless, the determination of capture was more complex than it might appear. A difference of 58% was noticed between the lowest threshold of 66 mA and the highest of 104 mA, and one subject tended to develop tachycardia. This happened in response to discomfort, which was similar with all the devices. Furthermore, it is possible that some subjects were incorrectly evaluated as having experienced capture when the native rhythm matched the pacing rate, but this could not be established by devices that were used without monitoring. Manual pulse palpation proved difficult due to skeletal muscle contraction, and the use of pulse oximetry in such cases may be misleading. As the range of current was not the same for all the devices, increasing the mean capture threshold either gradually or by large increments of 50, 100, or 150 mA did not provide reliable information. Finally, the discomfort appeared to exhibit large intersubject and intrasubject variability, and the authors had no explanation for the differences observed.

Another feature that varies in the different pacing devices concerns the surface area of the electrodes. We know that there is a negative relation between the active electrode surface and the capture threshold. Thus, Zoll et al.[8] found that threshold decreased rapidly when the area of the electrode increased up to 12 cm^2, and then more slowly up to 50 cm^2 (<1 mA/cm^2). In a concomitant study, the pain threshold was also expressed in terms of current density. For an electrode area of 25 cm^2 and more, this threshold was less than 2 mA/cm^2, and remained stable when the electrode area increased.

Until now, a high impedance gel was generally used for transcutaneous cardiac stimulation. One might think that tolerance changes with gel impedance. Thus Heller et al.[12] conducted a large study comprising 30 volunteers with 16 pacer/pad combinations to determine whether or not tolerance depends on gel electrode impedance. The mean threshold current was 99 ± 10 mA, and they found no significant variation for the pain scores which were 5.8 and 4.9, respectively, for low and high impedance gel electrodes.

In some studies, the threshold current was found to drop significantly in one of several electrode positions evaluated in the same subject by moving the anterior electrode on the left precordium. Meibom et al.,[13] who used this method in healthy humans, in a relaxed situation, found a mean threshold of 50 mA. Nevertheless, despite this low threshold, one subject left his bed because of strong painful knocks on the chest. The discomfort appeared to be dependent on large intersubject and intrasubject variability, even though the same device, and gel and electrode area, were the same for all subjects.

In an emergency department, capture with pulse could not be obtained in patients because of electromechanical dissociation, asystole and intolerable discomfort at 70 mA, whereas spontaneous bradycardia was well tolerated. This happened in 3/26 patients in the study of Dunn et al.[14] Of the remaining patients, 35% reported severe discomfort. Pain was observed to be severe at a threshold ranging from 40 to 110 mA, and intolerable at 40 to 70 mA. All the patients concerned were under 70 years old. Discomfort did not seem related to the capture threshold, but nevertheless intensified when it had to be raised.

NTCP has constituted an alternative therapy for some patients for whom transvenous pacing was contraindicated because of thrombolytic therapy or right acute myocardial infarct complicated by bradycardia. Complications caused by temporary transvenous pacemakers have led to renewed interest in NTCP. Thus, in 13/28 patients with acute myocardial infarction, Worley et al.[15] observed a mean capture threshold of 67.2 mA (range: 48 to 90 mA), combined with success for resuscitative measures. However, a 97-year-old woman with torsades de pointe, possibly due to interference with a permanent pacemaker failure, could not be paced, even at 140 mA. Nevertheless, this study showed that NTCP could be applied with success in cases of few residual viable myocardium. NTCP can also be satisfactory when drugs have no effect. In right ventricular infarction, Little[16] observed that external cardiac pacing increased the heart rate and led to marked hemodynamic improvement, whereas running wide open infusion of isoproterenol had no effect on the heart rate.

Tolerance depends on factors directly due to the patient's condition and displays great unexplained variability. As regards tolerance of the proposed devices, too many parameters appear to interact and have not been explored individually. At present, it is not possible to establish which parameter is the most important. This discussion does not concern the use of NTCP in emergency situations that require pacing, regardless of the necessary current amplitude. When the patient regains consciousness, tolerance can be a problem, for example, during transport to an intensive care unit.

Pacing Threshold Evaluation

The threshold value is the current amplitude inducing electrical capture shown on the ECG record by a QRS complex of 120 msec or more following the stimulation artefact, usually with an inverse large T wave. The electrogram resembles that of a ventricular extrasystole. When electrical capture happens, palpable pulses are expected during the following five or ten minutes. Threshold is usually expressed in milliamperes (mA), corresponding to the imposed current. Allowing for the area pad with negative polarity (i.e., the active electrode), the value can be given in mA/cm^2 and termed the current density. In many studies, the surface area of the electrodes was not mentioned and current density could therefore not be calculated.

None of the human or experimental studies reviewed enabled us to obtain a mean pacing threshold value with a normal range, even for a particular device with a stable duration of stimulation, or for the same duration using different devices. Furthermore, in most of the publications, the electrode pads were stated to have high impedance, but no value was indicated. The position, number, size of the electrodes, and wave form of the impulse might explain the differences between the current threshold amplitudes reported, but these parameters were not always indicated.

This chapter deals only with the results obtained in clinical and experimental studies with one pair of electrodes. Usually, they were located in an antero-posterior (AP) or latero-lateral (LL) position when the heart was situated in the left hemithorax. The preferred placement of the active electrode was somewhere around the apex.

For endovenous cardiac stimulation, antiarrhythmic drugs are known to lower the pacing threshold, and the same might apply with NTCP. According to Klein et al.,[17], the mean external pacing threshold was 88 mA (range: 80 to 100 mA) and was lower (75 ± 7 mA) but not significantly different in patients on antiarrhythmic drugs.

With NTCP, the value for this threshold in adults was sometimes as low as 20 mA. However, the conditions under which the method was applied to these cases were not examined by the authors. This was found in the study by Prochaczek et al.[18] who used the method in hospital with symmetrical AP positioning of the electrodes (V_3) in normal patients (mean ventricular threshold of 59 mA). The same minimum threshold was found by Dunn et al.[14] in an emergency department on patients with pulses.

In both these studies, the current threshold range was wide, and one might think that the use of a high current threshold would induce more vigorous contraction. In fact, Altamura et al.,[19] who obtained a mean ventricular threshold of 74 ± 14 mA (1.48 mA/cm^2), found different sites of myocardial activation, depending on the current amplitude. In an effort to induce atrial capture, they obtained it with 138 ± 25 mA (2.76 mA/cm^2). Then, after an 86% rise in current amplitude, the atria were paced preferentially to the ventricles, although they were located more posteriorly with the same sagittal axis of current flow. When simultaneous atrial and ventricular pacing occurred, this stimulus was confined to the interval between the end of the refractoriness and the beginning of the next ventricular depolarization. One wonders whether other studies with a high threshold obtained atrial activation but not ventricular capture. If atrial and ventricular contractions occur, NTCP should also perhaps be used for noninvasive determination of simple electrophysiological parameters such as sinus node recovery time. To analyze correctly what happens, ECG records must not have any artefact on the base line.

Most studies in man have so far concerned adults and very few have been conducted in children. As the child's thorax is smaller, it would be normal to have a lower current threshold, using adult electrodes. According to Beland et al.,[20] who studied 22 anesthetized young subjects aged 11 months to 18 years, the threshold was 63 ± 14 mA (range: 42 to 98 mA) using adult electrodes, i.e., similar to the postanesthetic threshold in adults, and 51 ± 11 mA (range: 29 to 82 mA) with small electrodes. Current densities for the adult and smaller electrode were respectively 0.8 mA/cm^2 and 7.2 mA/cm^2. The authors proposed the use of smaller electrodes (diameter about 3 cm) for these patients, especially when they weighed less than 15 kg (33 lbs). Furthermore, they found that current density and energy requirements did not vary with age (from 0.9 to 17.9 years), weight (from 6.96 to 51 kg), or chest size.

In the study by Beland et al., the absence of correlations between current threshold and patient morphology was surprising. This was also reported by Delhumeau et al.[21] in 33 adults during general anesthesia. No correlation was found between threshold current and weight (67 ± 10 kg), chest diameter (20 ± 2 cm) or heart/chest ratio (0.53 ± 0.07). These authors confirm that the position of the electrodes is very important. Surprisingly, in their anesthetized patients,[21] the mean threshold current was 110 mA (range: 85 to 150 mA), i.e., higher than in previous studies, and current density was 1.4 mA/cm².

Berliner et al.,[22] on the contrary, reported a threshold current in 21 normal patients which may have been affected by their age (20–75 years) and by chest size. Its mean value was 142 ± 57 mA. These findings could not be interpreted because with their NTCP device, the current jumped from 50 to 100 and then 200 mA, with no intermediate value. In regard to heart size, the relation with threshold current was slightly or not significant.

Echocardiography in the left lateral decubitus position which Madsen et al.[23] used, the heart is near the anterior precordium, not far from the apical electrode patch. In a study of myocardial activation, they found a low threshold, from 38 to 78 mA (0.51 to 0.93 mA/cm²), in ten healthy volunteers aged from 23 to 33 years.

Other correlations have been explored: according to Kelley et al.[24] who studied all the above demographic data in 23 patients in sinus rhythm having undergone a cardiopulmonary bypass, weight (75 ± 13 kg), ischemic time (61 ± 32 mn), and body surface area (1.85 ± 0.20 m²) were not related to an increase in current threshold, especially at closed chest time, and only increased cardiac output (4.54 ± 1.05 vs 5.73 ± 1.34 l/mn) and core temperature (36.05 ± 0.54 vs 37.35 ± 0.59°C) were correlated with a statistically significant increase in this threshold. Advancing age (59 ± 11 years old) and pump time (131 ± 46 mn) were of borderline significance. In these cases, the influence of hypothermia, myocardial edema, hemopericardium, biological events, hypoxia, pericardial, and mediastinal air can be suggested.

So far, NTCP has been used to treat bradycardia as well as tachycardia. Taking into account the diagrammatic representation of Coumel's original technique,[25] the ability of NTCP to pace the atria and ventricles simultaneously could be useful in reentrant supraventricular tachycardia and reciprocating AV junctional tachycardia.

Recently, NTCP was also used for programmed ventricular stimulation with single or multiple extrastimuli. Triggered by a spontaneous beat of the tachycardia, this method was used for tachycardia termination, but required devices with a large scale of paced rhythms and separate programming of the intervals between the stimuli. The application of endovenous modalities to tachycardia termination might be possible with NTCP. Luck et al.[26] have used this method to terminate sustained VT morphologies. The mean ventricular threshold was 60 mA after lidocaine (5 mg/kg, 200 mg) in demand ventricular mode (likened to VVI mode) for a VT of 180 ppm in a 76-year-old woman, and 42 mA in asynchronous ventricular mode (likened to VOO mode) for a VT of 150 ppm in a 43-year-old woman. In 88% of induced VT morphologies,[27] external burst pacing terminated VT with a pacing cycle length of 282 ± 44 msec vs 298 ± 93 msec with endocardial pacing. In one patient, there was an acceleration of tachycardia.

A similar acceleration was terminated by NTCP in the study by Grubb et al.[28] In this field too, the range of threshold current was large. In sustained ventricular tachycardia during subsequent episodes of monophasic VT at 145 ppm, overdrive pacing (200 pm) with 120 mA resulted in the termination of all VT.

One question to be considered concerns the possible risk of ventricular arrhythmia connected with high threshold current. In six normal dogs, Voorhees et al.[29] determined a safety factor using a sutured active stainless steel electrode located centrally over the site requiring the lowest pacing current, using low resistive gel. This factor was calculated from the ratio of threshold stimulation to induced threshold fibrillation (using the same electrode). The safety factor was never less than 7 and averaged 12.6 for impulse durations of 1 to 50 msec. The pacing threshold was 70 mA but the calculated current density was high (9.2 mA/cm^2), as the negative electrode was small.

In dogs with A-V block or normal sinus rhythm, the safety factor for VT and VF was found by Zoll et al.[8] to have a mean value of 9 ± 2 (range: 5 to 12.5) for stimuli durations of 2 to 100 msec.

These results were obtained in normal dogs. In an emergency situation involving humans, this safety factor should be modified. In view of the risk of known or unknown associated pathology, the asynchronous ventricular mode (VOO) cannot be used but must be replaced by demand ventricular mode (VVI).

Electrode Positioning

Hemodynamic and electrophysiological studies of the threshold incidence of site, area, impedance electrodes, number or duration of pulses, and shape of current are easier to conduct in animals. Energy consumption is mainly determined by the positioning of the electrodes.

Geddes et al.[30] defined a precordial "pacing window" to identify the region with the lowest current threshold. This approach needed mapping with a 1 cm diameter electrode (cathode), paired with a stable electrode in the LL position. The mean threshold in 18 anesthetized dogs was 34.3 mA (10.9 mA/cm^2). This study was performed to determine that little was to be gained with an active electrode larger than 5 cm in diameter.

Although the threshold value is mainly determined by the location and to some extent by the number of the electrodes, no anatomical study has been performed to evaluate their optimal location and number. This seems to be due to the presence of lung, muscles, bones, and skin which deviate the current in different ways in each individual's geometry before reaching the heart. How to determine promptly the best arrangement of the electrodes in a given situation has not yet been found.

NTCP has been applied in bradycardia, normal rhythm, and tachycardia. Was the threshold different in each case, especially when a complete AV block occurred? In ten closed-chest chronic heart block dogs (53–62 ppm) in which bradycardia (33 ppm) was induced after lidocaine (bolus IV 50–100 mg and infusion of 3–4 mg/mn), Niemann et al.[31] found a high mean threshold of 130 mA (2.6 mA/cm^2) in latero-lateral (LL) electrode position and 160 mA (3.2 mA/cm^2) in the oropharyngeal-epigastrium (OE) position. Skeletal muscle contractions were obvious but less prominent in the LL than OE position, for comparable strengths. Mean arterial pressure, even under lidocaine, and cardiac output increased under LL external pacing, as with endovenous stimulation.

The site of application of stimulation may be assumed to give a current distribution which could reach the heart in different ways. In seven surgically prepared dogs with 128 simultaneous recording electrodes located on the atria, interventricular septum, subepicardium, and subendocardium of the left and right ventricles, Tang et al.[32] evaluated the activation pattern and incidence of electrode positioning in the AP, LL and right upper-left lower LL (RU/LL-LL) positions. The threshold current values were 70 mA (0.85 ± 0.43 mA/cm^2) in the AP position and 117 mA (1.43 ± 0.45 mA/cm^2) in the LL position with retrograde VA conduction. The ventricular sites of early activation were observed in anterior LV or RV in the AP position, and lateral RV in the LL position. Threshold current was 130 mA (1.59 ± 0.16 mA/cm^2) in the RU/LL-LL position with antegrade AV conduction at low current and with atrial and ventricular capture at high current.

In all these applications, the anterior electrode close to the myocardial mass might be negative, as the current density decreases with the square of the distance. This negative site should be located above the apex. In our experiments with four closed-chest anesthetized mongrel dogs (21 ± 3 kg), the negative patch (78 cm^2) was centered under fluoroscopy on the diaphragmatic region (D), 2 cm above the apex (A) or 4 cm above position A, corresponding in part to the left lung (L). The D, A, and L positions were located at various levels on the medial line of the left hemithorax. The right positive electrode (50 cm^2) was stable in the LL position, on the medial line of the right hemithorax, corresponding to the V_4R ECG level in humans. We used pregelled, self-adhesive electrode pads having a gel of high impedance controlled after each experiment with the electrodes face to face (677 ± 23 ohms under 60 ppm and 60 mA). The threshold measurement was based on both electrocardiographic and hemodynamic monitoring. The threshold was lower in A (58 mA, 0.74 ± 0.02 mA/cm^2), 91% higher in D (111 ± 6 mA), and 56% higher in L (91 ± 6 mA). In position D, simultaneous stimulation of respiratory rhythm occurred. Increasing the stimulus duration showed that the threshold did not change up to a duration of 10 msec in positions A and D, and up to more than 20 msec in position L. This study showed the importance of the choice of the negative site. We had the opportunity to use an X-ray view to know exactly the position of the ventricles. In emergency, a more practicable method should be found to locate the cardiac mass quickly and more precisely.

No systematic pharmacological study has been conducted to establish exactly which therapeutic drugs affect the application of NTCP. Some particular situations have concerned external cardiac pacing. Falk et al.[33] found that propranolol and verapamil have no significant effect on external threshold. Cummins et al.[34] reported than NTCP might be lifesaving for a 5-year-old girl after ingestion of yew plant leaves which possess transient cardiac toxicity and can produce fatal conduction disturbances. Threshold studies on the cardiac pacemaker indicate that physiological variables, pharmacological agents, and lead electrodes do affect NTCP as reported by Dohrmann et al.[35] These effects are superimposable for patients in emergency situations who have had previous cardiological treatments. This is why Sowton et al.[36] attributed the decrease or increase in pacing threshold to a day-to-day increase in sympathetic tone or a decrease in parasympathetic tone.

Previous clinical events may sometimes not be known to the paramedical unit in situations of symptomatic brady- or tachyarrhythmias. The location and size of the electrode and the choice of pulse duration are important in avoiding the risk of unsuccessful stimulation, and produce minimal skin sensation in conscious patients. In case of patient discomfort, low doses of sedative drugs can be given until arrival in hospital. As underlying tissues contain pain receptors, and motor and sensory nerve fibers, the law of stimulation means that more current is required if the pulse does not rise abruptly (process of accommodation). Because tissue properties are different and change with time, it is possible to optimize the ratio of pain threshold to pacing threshold by a judicious choice of pulse duration. Geddes et al.[37] showed from both theoretical considerations and experimental data that the choice of the optimum duration can minimize the stimulation of pain fibers and that in both cases the strength-duration curve had the same shape. This showed that the current must increase when duration decreases. The pacing curve lay above the pain curve. Optimal pulse duration minimizes skin pain and should be 10 msec or more. In an experimental study[38] in which the electrodes were positioned over the cardiac mass, we found that the increase in pulse duration to a value greater than 10 msec was not followed by a decrease of threshold when the electrodes were in the LL position. This was observed whether the polarity on the apical electrode was negative or positive.

Electrode Impedance and Gel Characteristics

In most studies, electrode impedance was high, contrary to that employed for external cardiac defibrillation. For standard gel-pad as well as metal-plate electrodes, a high density current is known to exist at the electrode periphery, and energy is not evenly distributed over the electrode surface. According to Kim et al.,[39] this high concentration of current density, combined with an increase in temperature, might be related to the site of pain and cause other lesions. In that case, other parameters should be used to minimize the threshold and give uniform current density. Resistivity, thickness, and width of the gel layer have been observed to interact with the most effective position. Using two different levels, each of which was a two-dimensional model of a cross-sectional body, Fahy et al.[40] found that the design of the electrodes did not affect the efficacy of defibrillation. For external stimulation, increasing gel resistivity eliminated the current borderline spikes, and simultaneous reduction of the diameter caused a rise in current density in the central portion of the plate electrode.

The results of these studies do not enable clear rules to be formulated. Consequently, the appropriate method of applying each pacing device must be found and each symptom or event in cardiopulmonary resuscitation care must be taken into account. This application has to allow for the specific parameters of each device and the differences among individual patients (stoutness, cardiac mass, and previous cardiac pathology or therapy).

In prehospital external pacing, an additional parameter has to be observed: the time-dependent success of NTCP. The treatment of asystole or electromechanical dissociation reported by Hedges, Barthell et al.[41,42] has had little success with NTCP, even if the mean advanced medical response time was as low as possible. This justifies the controversy concerning the beneficial effect of this method if used early after cardiac arrest, before any attempt at drug therapy, and concomitantly with cardiopulmonary resuscitation. When asystole fails to respond to standard drug therapy, it might be too late to improve survival with another method. NTCP has been recognized as a widely available method by the American Heart Association[43] in the treatment of bradycardia (Fig. 2). In symptomatic atrioventricular (AV) block, the procedure shown in Figure 2 has been developed for CPR treatment and emergency care, and should be completed by other nonspecified care such as chest thump. In case of ischemia, infarction, or hypotension with bradycardia, medical investigators should primarily use NTCP. As emergency mobile care units do not have the same guidelines in the USA and Europe, it needs specific recommendations. The time-dependent success of cardiac stimulation should be taken into account when elaborating solutions for advanced cardiac life support.

Conclusion

As already mentioned, previous electrophysiological studies have proved that the use of NTCP is beneficial. When tolerance is acceptable, this method could also help when the invasive method cannot be used repeatedly.

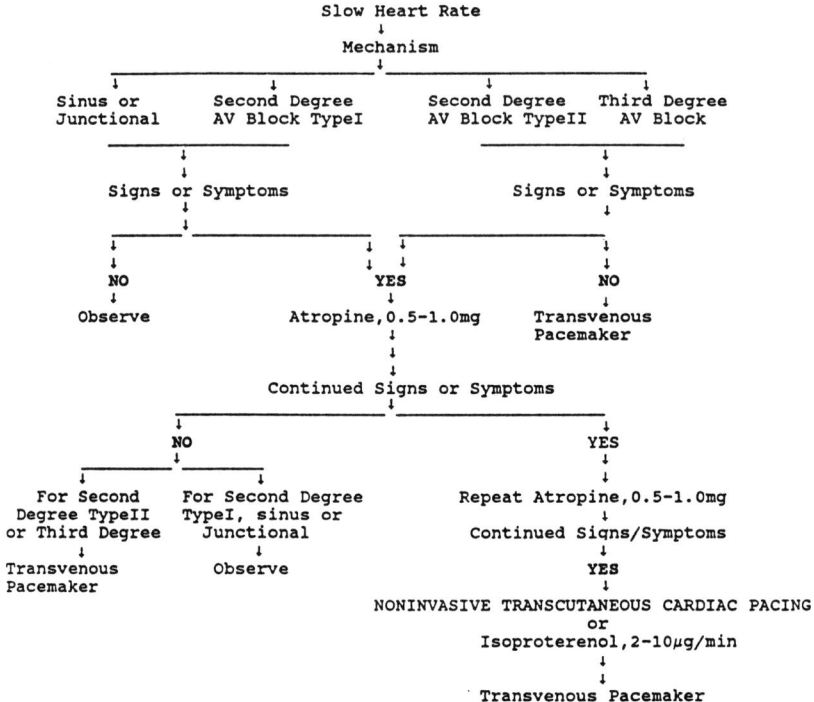

Figure 2: *Therapeutic algorithm for bradycardia (heart rate less than 60 ppm). Reproduced with permission. Textbook of Advanced Cardiac Life Support, 1987, 1990. Copyright American Heart Association.*

As regards tolerance, pacing rate, and threshold, two distinct applications of NTCP could be suggested:
• The first applies to mobile emergency medical care units, where the delay in intervention must be as brief as possible and where qualified and well-prepared medical staff can interpret the ECG and decide either to apply this method promptly during adapted CPR (ventilation and rewarming) or to administer drugs.[53] In the first case, a multifunction unit can stimulate and/or defibrillate and monitor the ECG during transport. Such a unit requires rheologic or mechanographic means of checking the hemodynamic efficacy of cardiac pacing. In this field, more studies are necessary to find an adequate

method of stimulation under various emergency conditions, with constant ECG monitoring and ventilation.

In this review, we have reported certain studies in detail to indicate the parameters for which a coordinated approach by medical staff and manufacturers could help to extend the use of NTCP, a safe and noninvasive method.

The second application could be in electrophysiological laboratories, which might provide better facilities for more extensive ranges of stimulation frequencies, modes of stimulation, and pulse duration, all of which require further evaluation. This area is new and may develop considerably if the firms concerned can produce devices adaptable to each case. Such devices do not need to be transportable because they will be used in operating rooms and on conscious patients during bed rest.

References

1. Duchenne De Boulogne: De l'électrisation localisée et de son application á la pathologie et á la thérapeutique. Paris, Bailliére Ed, 1872.
2. McWilliam JA: Electrical stimulation of the heart in man. Br Med J 1:348, 1889.
3. Zoll PM: Resuscitation of the heart in ventricular standstill by external electric stimulation. N Engl J Med 247:768, 1952.
4. Levy Solal E, Morin P, Zacouto F: Premiers résultats d'électrosystologie cardiaque. Sem des Hôpitaux de Paris, 29:10, 1953.
5. Donzelot E, Zacouto F, Coraboeuf E: L'entrainement électrosystolique. Ses applications cliniques. Arch des Mal du Coeur 48:362, 1955.
6. Furman S, Scwhedel J: An intracardiac pacemaker for Stokes-Adams seizures. N Engl J of Med 261:943, 1959.
7. Bouvrain Y, Zacouto F: Entraînement électro-systolique par électrodes intra-cavitaires au cours d'un syndrome d'Adams-Stockes. Soc Méd des Hôpt de Paris 4:105, 1961.
8. Zoll RH, Zoll PM, Belgard AH: Noninvasive cardiac stimulation. In: Cardiac Pacing: Electrophysiology and Pacemaker Technology. Feruglio GA (ed), Piccin Medical Books, Padova, 1983, p. 593.
9. Alferness CA, Tang ASL, Rollins DL, et al.: External pacing from multiple electrodes in dogs (abstract). PACE 14:337, 1991.
10. Zacouto F: Brevet Français 651 632. Perfectionnement aux appareils électro-médicaux. Demandé en 1953, accepté en 1960. Paris.
11. Heller MB, Peterson J, Ilkahpamipour K, et al.: A comparative study of five transcutaneous pacing devices in unanesthetized human volunteers. Prehosp and Disaster Med 4:15, 1989.
12. Heller MB, Mac Leod B, Yealy DM, et al.: The effect of different

combinations of external pacemakers and pads on pacing thresholds, capture rate and patient tolerance (abstract). Ann Emerg Med 17:1, 1988.
13. Meibom J, Vilhelmsen R, Madsen JK: A new noninvasive temporary pacemaker (Zoll-NTP). In: Cardiac Pacing. Gomez FP (ed). Editorial Grouz, Madrid, 1985, p. 397.
14. Dunn DL, Gregory JJ: Noninvasive temporary pacing: Experience in a community hospital. Heart and Lung 18:23, 1989.
15. Worley SJ, Bride WM: External transthoracic pacing in patients with acute myocardial infarction. In: Acute Coronary Care. Califf RM and Wagner GS (eds). Martinus Nijhoff Publishing, Boston, 1987.
16. Little T: External cardiac pacing. Ann Emerg Med 17:640, 1988.
17. Klein LS, Miles WM, Heger JJ, et al.: Transcutaneous pacing: patient tolerance, strength-interval relations and feasibility for programmed electrical stimulation. Amer J Cardiol 62:1126, 1988.
18. Prochaczek P, Galecka J: The effect of suppression of the distortion artifact during transcutaneous pacing on the shape of the QRS complex. PACE 13:2022, 1990.
19. Altamura G, Toscano S, Lo Bianco, et al.: Emergency cardiac pacing for severe bradycardia. PACE 13:2038, 1990.
20. Beland MJ, Hesslein PS, Finlay CD, et al.: Noninvasive transcutaneous cardiac pacing in children. PACE 10:1262, 1987.
21. Delhumeau A, Granry JC, Cocaud J, et al.: Détermination des seuils de stimulation cardiaque externe pendant l'anesthésie. Ann Fr Anesth Réanim 6:429, 1987.
22. Berliner D, Okun M, Peters RW, et al.: Transcutaneous temporary pacing in the operating room. JAMA 254:84, 1985.
23. Madsen K, Pedersen F, Grande P, et al.: Normal myocardial enzymes and normal echocardiographic findings during noninvasive transcutaneous pacing. PACE 13:1188, 1988.
24. Kelley JS, Royster RL, Angert KC, et al.: Efficacy of noninvasive transcutaneous cardiac pacing in patients undergoing cardiac surgery. Anesthesiology 70:747, 1989.
25. Coumel P, Cabrol C, Fabiato A, et al.: Tachycardie permanente par rythme réciproque. I. Preuves du diagnostic par stimulation auriculaire et ventriculaire. II. Traitement par l'implantation intracorporelle d'un stimulateur cardiaque avec entrainement simultané de l'oreillette et du ventricule. Arch Mal Coeur 60:1830, 1967.
26. Luck JC, Davis D: Termination of sustained tachycardia by external noninvasive pacing. PACE, 10:1125, 1987.
27. Luck JC, Grubb BP, Artman SE, et al.: Termination of sustained ventricular tachycardia by external noninvasive pacing. Am J Cardiol 61:574, 1988.
28. Grubb BP, Temesy-Armos P, Hahn H, et al.: The clinical use of external noninvasive pacing in the termination of sustained ventricular tachycardia. PACE 13:1092, 1990.
29. Voorhees WD, Foster KS, Geddes LA, et al.: Safety factor for precordial pacing: Minimum current threshold for pacing and for ventricular fibrillation by vulnerable-period stimulation. PACE 7:356, 1984.

30. Geddes LA, Voorhees WD, Babbs CF, et al.: Precordial pacing windows. PACE 7:806, 1984.
31. Niemann JT, Rosborough JP, Garner D, et al.: External noninvasive cardiac pacing: A comparative hemodynamic study of two techniques with conventional endocardial pacing. PACE 7:230, 1984.
32. Tang ASL, Derfus DL, Wharton JM, et al.: The effect of electrode location on activation sequence and threshold during external pacing. JACC, 11:(Abstr) 164A, 1988.
33. Falk RH, Knowlton AA, Battinelli NJ: The effect of propranolol and verapamil on external pacing threshold: A placebo-controlled study. PACE 11:1439, 1988.
34. Cummins RO, Haulman J, Quan L, et al.: Near-fatal yew berry intoxication treated with external cardiac pacing and digoxin-specific FAB antibody fragments. Ann Emerg Med 19:38, 1990.
35. Dohrmann ML, Goldslager NF: Myocardial stimulation threshold in patients with cardiac pacemakers: Effect of physiologic variables, pharmacologic agents, and lead electrodes. Cardiology Clinics 3:527, 1985.
36. Sowton E, Barr I: Physiological changes in threshold. Ann NY Acad Sci 167:679, 1969.
37. Geddes LA, Babbs CF, Voorhees WD, et al.: Choice of optimum pulse duration for precordial cardiac pacing: A theoretical study. PACE 8:862, 1985.
38. Birkui PJ, Trigano JA, Degonde J: Efficacité hémodynamique de la stimulation cardiaque transcutanée. Bull Acad Natle Méd 9:1361, 1990.
39. Kim Y, Fahy JB, Tupper BJ: Optimal electrode designs for electrosurgery, defibrillation, and external cardiac pacing. IEEE Trans Biomed Eng 33:845, 1986.
40. Fahy JB, Kim Y, Ananthaswamy A: Optimal electrode configurations for external cardiac pacing and defibrillation: An inhomogeneous study. IEEE Trans Biomed Eng 34:743, 1987.
41. Hedges JR, Syverud SA, Dalsey WC: Prehospital trial of emergency transcutaneous cardiac pacing. Circulation 76:1337, 1987.
42. Barthell E, Troiano P, Olson D, et al.: Prehospital external cardiac pacing: A prospective, controlled clinical trial. Ann Emerg Med 17:1221, 1988.
43. American Heart Association: Textbook of Advanced Cardiac Life Support. 1987–1990, p. 242.

II

Biological Aspects

Chapter 3

Myocardial Enzyme Monitoring Pacing

Jan Kyst Madsen, MD, DMSC

A single electrical discharge as part of a DC-conversion does not cause detectable rise in creatine kinase MB (CK-MB), indicating that the myocardium is not damaged.[1] Transcutaneous pacing uses much lower electrical currents but may still be detrimental as several discharges are used over a long period of time. Furthermore, it has been shown that repeated electrical discharges may cause myocardial necrosis if the time interval between is very short.[2] It is most important that the benefits obtained from noninvasive transcutaneous cardiac pacing (NTCP) are not outweighed by myocardial damage during the procedure. In the clinical studies using NTCP, there is only one case report indicating that the procedure does not affect the myocardium.[3] There are two major studies, one in man and the other in dogs, that have evaluated the possible myocardial damage of NTCP.

Canine Model

Syverud et al. performed 30 mn of NTCP on ten mongrel dogs.[4] These animals weighed 18 to 28 kg and were paced with 100 mA at a heart rate of 80 ppm.
Creatine kinase (CK) and creatine kinase myocardial band CK-

From *Noninvasive Transcutaneous Cardiac Pacing* edited by Pierre Birkui, M.D., Jacques Trigano, M.D., and Paul Zoll, M.D., © 1993, Futura Publishing Company, Inc., Mount Kisco, NY.

MB were determined from blood samples taken before, immediately after, and 2, 4, and 24 hours after pacing. The results of CK analysis are shown in Figure 1. An immediate fall right after pacing following by an increase at 2, 4, and 24 hours were observed. However, none of these changes were significant. There were no changes in CK-MB.

The changes in CK may reflect slight skeletal muscle damage, but there are no indications of myocardial damage, despite the fact that the electrical impulse during pacing is relatively larger in this study of dogs than the electrical stimulus used in humans. The impulse is 80 mA, but the animals' weights were only one-third that of adult humans. The results are further supported by the finding of a normal electrocardiogram after pacing.[4]

However, macroscopic examination revealed myocardial pallor, and microscopic examination revealed focal myofibril coagulation in

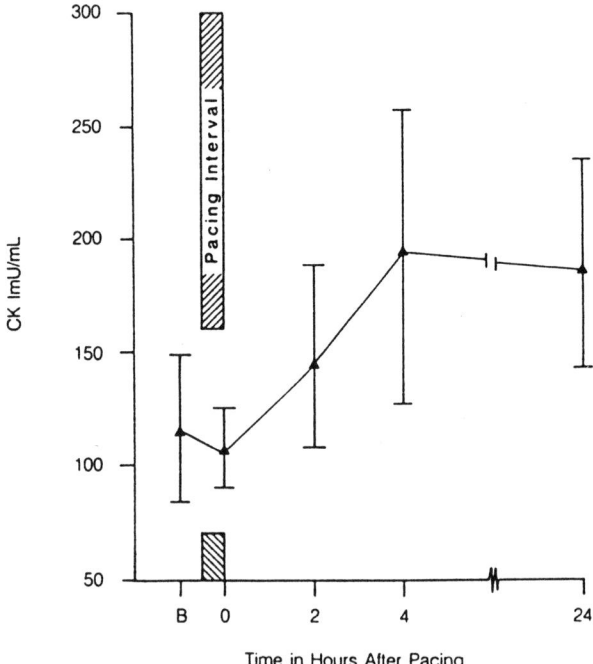

Figure 1. *Serum concentrations of creatine kinase (CK) before and after 30 mn of NTCP (mean ± SD). (Reproduced from Syverud SA et al.[3] with permission from the authors and the Annals of Emergency Medicine.)*

the right ventricular outflow tract and perivascular microinfarcts in the posterior left ventricular myocardium.[4,5] These changes are very small and are thought not to be of any clinical significance. Furthermore, the electrical stimulus in this study was approximately three times higher than the electrical stimulus used in humans.

Human Study

We examined the possible myocardial damage from NTCP in ten healthy volunteers.[6]

Material and Methods

Five men and five women ranging from 23 to 33 years of age participated. They weighed in median 71 kg, range 52 to 87 kg.

The electrodes were placed in the usual manner, with a negative front electrode of 75 cm^2 and a back electrode of 115 cm^2. We used a battery operated NTCP pacemaker, model 2011, manufactured by S&W Medico Teknik A/S, Denmark. The pulse duration was 40 msec. The subjects were paced during 30 mn. The pace rate was initially set 10%-20% above the resting heart rate, and gradually increased until 100% capture was achieved. The pace rate was from 85 to 115 ppm. The threshold for 100% capture was from 38 to 70 mA with a median of 59 mA. Two of the volunteers had significant discomfort, two others volunteers coughed frequently during pacing. Venous blood samples were drawn from the antecubital vein prior to pacing, immediately after and 1, 2, 3, 4, 6, 8, and 24 hours after pacing. The serum was stored at -20° C until the end of our study so that all samples from all volunteers could be analyzed together. Myoglobin[7] and the following enzymes were determined: creatine phosphokinase, creatinekinase MB, and lactate dehydrogenase.[8,9]

Results

The results are shown in Figure 2. There were absolutely no significant changes either in myoglobin or in any of the enzymes. The usual sex difference of CK was seen.

Lactate dehydrogenase, total creatine kinase, and myoglobin are

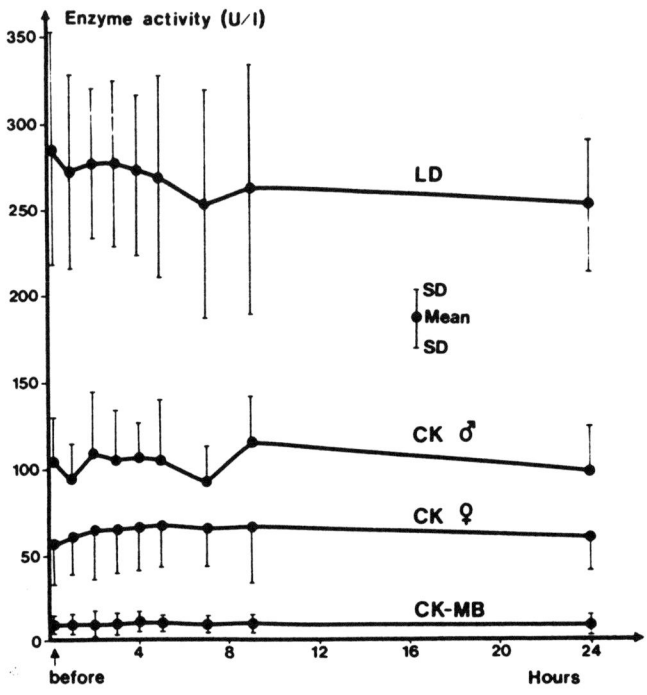

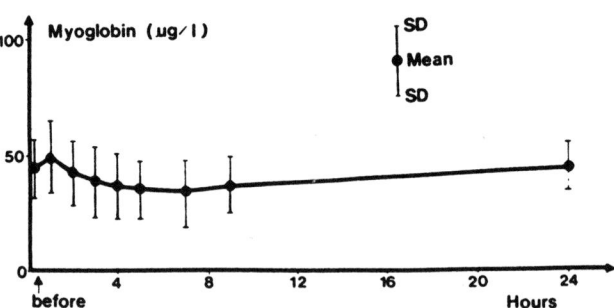

Figure 2. Serum concentrations of lactate dehydrogenase, creatine kinase, myoglobine, and creatine kinase MB before and after 30 mn of NTCP in 10 humans. (Reproduced from Madsen JK et al. with permission.[6])

very sensitive markers of both skeletal muscle and myocardial necrosis though not specific for myocardial tissue. CK-MB is almost only found in the myocardium and it is released into the blood and is a very sensitive marker of myocardial damage.[10] We did not see any significant changes in any of the enzymes or in myoglobin. This indicates that not even minor injuries occurred in the skeletal chest wall muscles or the myocardium during 30 mn NTCP.

Discussion and Conclusion

The above studies indicate that NTCP does not cause significant injury either to the myocardium or to the skeletal muscles; at least not for periods of NTCP up to 30 mn. NTCP for longer periods is rarely used. The studies are experimental in dogs and in healthy humans; however, there is reason to believe it will be different in patients.

Conclusions

As a consequence of the above considerations, it is reasonable to conclude that NTCP does not cause clinical damage either to the skeletal muscles or to the myocardium.

References

1. Neumeier D, Prellwits W, Knedel M: Differential diagnostic value of CK-MB activity measurements. *In*: Scient Meet Int Soc Clin Enzymol. Karger, London-Basel, 1977, p. 164.
2. Dahl CF, Ewy GA, Warner ED, et al.: Myocardial necrosis from direct current countershock. Effect of paddle electrode size and time interval between discharges. Circulation 50:956, 1974.
3. Clinton JE, Zoll PM, Zoll RH, et al.: Emergency noninvasive external cardiac pacing. J Emerg Med 2:155, 1984.
4. Syverud SA, Dalsey WC, Hedges JR, et al.: Transcutaneous cardiac pacing: Determination of myocardial injury in a canine model. An Emerg Med 12:745, 1983.
5. Kicklighter EJ, Syverud SA, Dalsey WC, et al.: Pathological aspects of transcutaneous cardiac pacing. Am J Emerg Med 3:108, 1985.
6. Madsen K, Pedersen F, Grande P, et al.: Normal myocardial enzymes and normal echocardiographic findings during noninvasive transcutaneous pacing. PACE 11:1188, 1988.

7. Rosano TG, Kenny MA: A radioimmunoassay for human serum myoglobin: Method development and normal values. Clin Chem 23:69, 1977.
8. The Committee on Enzymes of The Scandinavian Society for Clinical Chemistry and Clinical Physiology: Recommended method for determination of four enzymes in blood. Scan J Clin Lab Invest 33:290, 1973.
9. Grande P, Christiansen C: Clinical evaluation of different principles of CK-MB determination. Scan J Clin Lab Invest 43:197, 1983.
10. Grande P, Christiansen C, Pedersen A, et al.: Optimal diagnosis in acute myocardial infarction. Circulation 61:723, 1980.

III
Hemodynamic Studies

Chapter 4

The Hemodynamics of External Cardiac Pacing

Peter Schulman, MD, FACC

Although external cardiac pacing was introduced nearly four decades ago,[1] surprisingly few investigators have examined the hemodynamic effects of external cardiac pacing. Given the expanded application of older noninvasive techniques and the development of newer methods such as transesophageal echocardiography, the paucity of hemodynamic data on external cardiac pacing is all the more surprising. This chapter summarizes the limited number of clinical and experimental studies, both invasive and noninvasive, that have investigated hemodynamic effects of external cardiac pacing.

Measurements of Cardiac Pressures and Outputs during External Pacing

In the first hemodynamic study of external pacing in human subjects, Feldman et al.[2] recorded intracardiac pressures during external pacing in 16 patients who were undergoing diagnostic cardiac catheterization for coronary artery disease. Subjects were externally paced at increasing rates up to 85% of their maximal predicted heart rate. At the highest pacing rates all subjects, including the three without coronary artery disease, registered a rise in the right atrial

From *Noninvasive Transcutaneous Cardiac Pacing* edited by Pierre Birkui, M.D., Jacques Trigano, M.D., and Paul Zoll, M.D., © 1993, Futura Publishing Company, Inc., Mount Kisco, NY.

pressure, the pulmonary artery pressure, and the aortic pressure. Overall, there was a small decline in systemic resistance, and no significant change in cardiac index compared to the nonpaced state. Left ventricular end diastolic pressure (LVEDP) rose in all patients during pacing. However, in the coronary patients who developed angina during rapid pacing, the rise in LVEDP was greater, and the elevation persisted longer after pacing was discontinued.[2]

In our University of Connecticut study, Talit et al.[3] applied cardiac Doppler to study the hemodynamic effects of external cardiac pacing in ten adults free of coronary artery disease with normal left ventricular function. Doppler echocardiography was used to determine the changes in stroke volume and cardiac output induced by external pacing. In order to minimize the effect of altering the heart rate, the study subjects were paced at a rate as close as possible to their own heart rate. At a pacing rate 13% higher on average than the baseline sinus rate, left ventricular stroke volume was 24% lower compared to that during normal sinus rhythm. However, the faster heart rate during pacing partly compensated for the fall in stroke volume, so that average cardiac output fell only 14%.

The study of Talit[3] was the first to apply Doppler derived measurements of cardiac output to the investigation of the hemodynamics of external pacing (Fig. 1). The validity of this method has been well established.[4] Cardiac Doppler is readily available, easily performed, and entirely noninvasive. It is particularly well suited to study relative changes in cardiac stroke volume and cardiac output. In addition, the Doppler derived measurement of cardiac output has theoretical advantages over the Fick method for the determination of cardiac output, since the Fick method is influenced by oxygen consumption, which can increase because of pectoralis muscle contractions induced by external pacing.[2] Thus, Doppler echocardiography may be the method of choice to compare the effects of the various pacing modalities on cardiac output.

In another study comparing two methods of transvenous pacing, Belefer et al.[5] reported results analogous to those of Talit et al. Left ventricular stroke volume was 22% lower during ventricular pacing than during atrial pacing at the same rate.[5] A more recent case study also reported a 22% decline in stroke volume index when the pacing was changed from the (endocardial) AV sequential mode to external

The Hemodynamics of External Cardiac Pacing

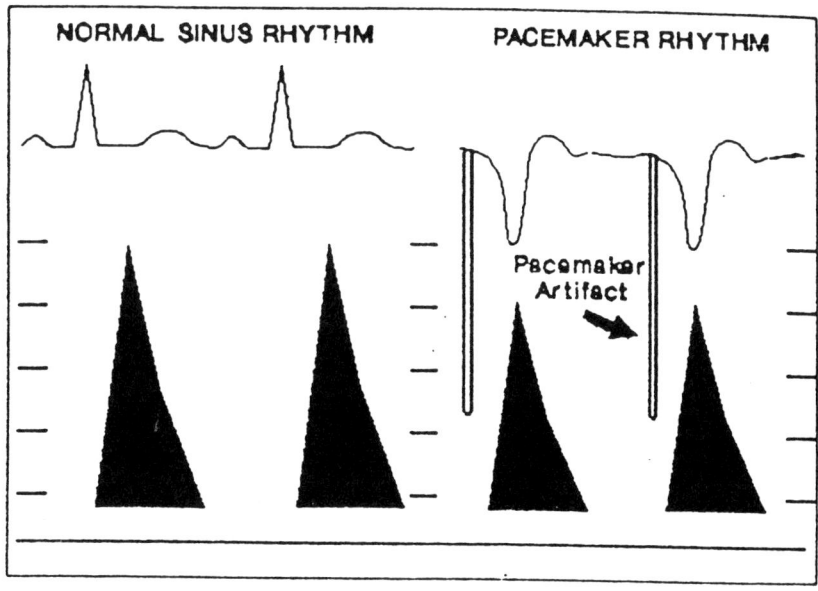

Figure 1. *Schematic representation of a continuous-wave Doppler tracing of aortic outflow. The velocity of blood flow is reflected on the vertical axis, and time is reflected on the horizontal axis. Sets of hatch marks appear every second, and marks are separated by 0.2 msec vertically. The first two beats represent the Doppler velocity integral of aortic outflow during normal sinus rhythm. The third and fourth beats reflect the smaller (by about 20%) velocity integral that occurs after the onset of external pacing.*

pacing.[6] These data suggest that the loss of atrioventricular (AV) synchrony accounts for the fall in cardiac output during external and ventricular endocardial pacing in comparison to sinus rhythm or "physiological" pacing.

Finally, in a recent literature survey, Baig and Perrins reviewed nine transvenous pacing studies that investigated the atrial contribution to cardiac output. For the most part, the subjects of these studies were patients with high grade heart block who had lost AV synchrony. In concordance with our data,[3] these studies showed that when AV synchrony was restored by atrial pacing, cardiac index rose anywhere from 10% to 22%.[7]

Sequence of Chamber Activation during External Pacing

In view of the hemodynamic benefits that accrue with the maintenance of atrioventricular synchrony, it would be ideal if the application of external pacing could result in a "normal" sequence of chamber activation. Relatively few studies have investigated the sequence of activation of the cardiac chambers during external pacing. Unfortunately, these studies demonstrate that atrioventricular synchrony does not occur with this type of pacing.

Varghese et al.[8] compared the activation sequence during external and ventricular endocardial pacing in six anesthetized dogs. Simultaneous intracardiac electrocardiograms and pressure measurements were recorded in the dogs' atria and ventricles during both methods of pacing. During external cardiac pacing, atria and ventricles were activated simultaneously. During endocardial pacing however, activation spread sequentially from the site of activation. Despite the different sequences of chamber activation of the two types of pacing, the resulting ventricular systolic pressures that were generated were not significantly different.[8]

In humans, only a limited number of studies have examined the sequence of chamber activation during external pacing. Eight normal volunteers were externally paced in a study by Falk et al.,[9] while an esophageal lead recorded atrial and ventricular electrograms. In contrast to the results in dogs,[8] the authors found that in humans, external pacing stimulates the ventricle first, and that the atrium was often activated in a retrograde fashion. The different results in dogs and humans are likely due to the different thoracic configurations found in these two species, or to the higher pacemaker outputs used by Varghese et al. or to both of these factors.[8,9]

Altamura et al.[10] reported similar results. Eight subjects were paced externally while endocardial electrodes recorded right atrial and ventricular activation. At lower energy pacemaker outputs that were tolerable to the study subjects, the majority of them had only ventricular activation with retrograde atrial activation through the AV node. However, by sedating the subjects and using otherwise intolerably high pacemaker energy outputs, simultaneous atrial and ventricular capture could be induced in four of eight subjects. Although simultaneous atrial and ventricular activation may not be useful for the temporary treatment of bradyarrhythmias, it may have a role in the termination of tachyarrhythmias.

In the hemodynamic study of Feldman et al.[2] discussed earlier in this chapter, the sequence of activation of the cardiac chambers was not assessed by intracardiac or esophageal electrocardiograms. However in six patients, continuous, simultaneous pressure recordings from the right and left ventricles at the onset of external pacing were performed. During external pacing, right ventricular pressure rose prior to left ventricular pressure, supporting the conclusion that the right ventricle is the first chamber to be activated by external pacing. However in their illustration, there is an apparent A wave on the right ventricular pressure curve preceding right ventricular systole;[2] this leads to some uncertainty over the sequence of chamber activation found.

Conclusion

Because of the paucity of studies that have investigated the hemodynamic effects of external cardiac pacing, only limited data are available (Table 1). Based upon the few published studies, it can be concluded that in human subjects, external pacing results in primarily ventricular activation. During pacing, intracardiac pressures rise. Left ventricular stroke volume is reduced approximately 20% to 25%, probably owing to the loss of atrioventricular synchrony. Increasing the pacing rate can partially restore the cardiac output closer to normal levels. In the future, a wider application of newer, noninva-

Table 1. Summary of Known Hemodynamic Effects of External Cardiac Pacing Compared to Normal Sinus Rhythm

1. Ventricular activation with variable retrograde atrial activation (If higher energy outputs are employed, simultaneous ventricular and atrial activation may occur).
2. Loss of atrioventricular synchrony.
3. Small elevations in atrial, ventricular, aortic and pulmonary pressures, and a slight fall in systemic vascular resistance.
4. 20% to 25% fall in left ventricular stroke volume.
5. A variable fall in cardiac output, depending upon the pacing rate.

sive testing methods will set the stage for a broader understanding of the hemodynamic consequences of external cardiac pacing.

References

1. Zoll PM, Ross RH, Belgard AH: External noninvasive electric stimulation of the heart. Crit Care Med 9: 393, 1981.
2. Feldman MD, Zoll PM, Aroesty JM, et al.: Hemodynamic response to noninvasive external cardiac pacing. Am J Med 84:395, 1988.
3. Talit U, Leach CN, Werner MS, et al.: The effect of external cardiac pacing on stroke volume. PACE 13:598, 1990.
4. Huntsman LL, Stewart DK, Barnes SR, et al.: Noninvasive determination of cardiac output in man. Circulation 67:593, 1983.
5. Befeler B, Hildner FJ, Javier RP, et al.: Cardiovascular dynamics during coronary sinus, right atrial, and right ventricular pacing. Am Heart J 81:372, 1971.
6. Trigano JA, Remond JM, Mourot F, et al.: Left ventricular pressure measurement during noninvasive transcutaneous cardiac pacing. PACE 12:1717, 1989.
7. Baig MW, Perrins EJ: The hemodynamics of cardiac pacing: Clinical and physiological aspects. Prog Cardiovasc Dis 33:283, 1991.
8. Varghese PJ, Bren G, Ross A: Electrophysiology of external pacing: A comparative study with endocardial pacing. Circulation (Suppl II) 66:349, 1982.
9. Falk RH, Ngai ST, Kumaki DJ, et al.: Cardiac activation during external cardiac pacing. PACE 10:503, 1987.
10. Altamura G, Toscano S, Bianconi L, et al.: Transcutaneous cardiac pacing: evaluation of cardiac activation. PACE 13:2017, 1991.

IV

Emergency Management

Chapter 5

Transcutaneous Cardiac Pacing in Cardiac Arrest

William C. Dalsey, MD, FACEP

Transcutaneous pacing was introduced into clinical practice in the United States by Dr. Paul Zoll and in England by Dr. Aubrey Leatham during the early 1950s.[1-4] They were able to successfully use transcutaneous pacing to restore a regular heart rhythm in patients with Stokes-Adam's attacks. Clinical use of transcutaneous pacing was also successful in temporarily treating other severe bradydysrhythmias as well as overdrive pacing ventricular and supraventricular tachydysrhythmias.

These early pacing systems used narrow pulse widths (2 msec) and small electrodes. The high voltage electrical pulses required for effective capture resulted in severe pain, muscle contractions, and skin burns. While transcutaneous pacing was demonstrated to successfully restore a regular heart rhythm temporarily, there was no permanent pacing system available. Transcutaneous pacing was not widely adopted.

Transvenous and transthoracic invasive pacing systems eliminated the problem of pain, burns, and muscle contractions and replaced transcutaneous pacing for all indications. Invasive cardiac pacing was not routinely advocated as a first line treatment in cardiac arrests. Invasive pacing was difficult, time consuming, expensive, and limited to physicians comfortable with these procedures. Gener-

From *Noninvasive Transcutaneous Cardiac Pacing* edited by Pierre Birkui, M.D., Jacques Trigano, M.D., and Paul Zoll, M.D., © 1993, Futura Publishing Company, Inc., Mount Kisco, NY.

ally, the use of invasive cardiac pacing during cardiac arrest was not found to be of significant benefit. Nevertheless, invasive cardiac pacing was attempted in asystole and bradydysrhythmias after pharmacologic therapy was ineffective. Occasional anecdotal and sporadic case reports described rare cases in which cardiac pacing appeared to be lifesaving. The general clinical attitude towards cardiac pacing in cardiac arrest was to attempt pacing when there was nothing else left to try. It was routinely unsuccessful.

Transcutaneous pacing was simultaneously reintroduced into clinical practice by several independent investigators in the mid 1980s.[5-10] They succeeded in improving the technique by widening the pulse width (20 msec) and enlarging the skin electrodes so that much smaller energies could be used.[7,11,12] This decrease in voltage significantly reduced pain and muscle contractions, and eliminated skin burns.

Safety and Efficacy

Initially, the updated transcutaneous pacing systems were used in cardiac arrest patients to prove their safety and efficacy.[13-19] Transcutaneous pacing was used in bradyasystolic cardiac arrests after pharmacological therapy failed. These studies demonstrated the safety and efficacy of transcutaneous pacing.[20-22] In fact, transcutaneous pacing was shown to result in electrical and mechanical capture twice as often as transvenous cardiac pacing. Electrical capture rates of 40% and mechanical capture rates of 20% were reported when transcutaneous pacing was used late in cardiac arrest resuscitation. Theoretically, the improved capture rates over transvenous pacing occur because transcutaneous pacing does not rely on an intact conduction system nor pinpoint positioning of the electrodes. With transcutaneous pacing, the entire myocardium appears to contract simultaneously. Restoration of effective cardiac output was established by several investigators.[23,24] Nevertheless, these clinical studies confirmed the dismal prognosis for bradyasystolic arrest despite the use of cardiac pacing when used late in the resuscitation.

The possibility of myocardial damage from the cumulative effect of repeated electrical pulses was investigated in animal models. These studies reported clinically insignificant damage when used for short periods.[21,22] The long-term cumulative effect from prolonged transcutaneous pacing has not been definitively investigated.

Groups led by Drs. Zoll and Syverud[19,20,24] noted some survivors when transcutaneous pacing was used early in the course of resuscitation. They reported some successful resuscitations when used within the first five minutes. Theoretically, the use of cardiac pacing to restore a normal functioning heart rhythm needs to occur before irreversible cellular damage results. Inadequate cellular oxygenation and blood flow can result in cell death after several minutes. All known resuscitation techniques are time-dependent, and success varies with their early application and restoration of a normal physiological state. In ventricular fibrillation, the success of defibrillation is time-dependent and approaches zero after ten minutes. Transcutaneous pacing in cardiac arrest is unlikely to be successful after ten minutes. Subsequent studies in cardiac arrests have focused on the early use of transcutaneous pacing as the first line treatment. Studies to determine if transcutaneous pacing may prove beneficial within the first few minutes of cardiac arrest have not been adequately performed. The difficulty in conducting this type of demanding trial may prevent this question from being definitively answered.

Caution should be expressed concerning patients with significant bradycardias related to hypoxia and airway compromise. Certainly, the resuscitation of these patients must begin with obtaining an adequate airway and ventilation. Frequently, restoration of adequate ventilation results in an increased heart rate. When the bradycardic rhythm persists, transcutaneous pacing or atropine may be useful in accelerating the heart rate.

Prearrest Indications

Indications for transcutaneous pacing include prearrest conditions which are anticipated to deteriorate into full cardiac arrest, refractory bradydysrhythmias, hemodynamically compromised bradydysrhythmias, overdrive pacing for selected tachydysrhythmias, and cardiac arrest. Once cardiac arrest actually occurs, the use of cardiac pacing has limited value. Studies have not demonstrated any statistically significant improvement in recovery from asystole with the use of transcutaneous cardiac pacing. Some evidence that early pacing in bradycardic arrest may alter morbidity and mortality needs further confirmation. However, in light of the relative safety of the technique and minimal success of other treatment modalities, it seemed reasonable to advocate its early use in bradycardic arrests. It is now recommended by the American Heart Association for use in bradycardic arrests. Premorbid conditions or those which are known to deteriorate into more malignant rhythms represent a use for transcutaneous pacing in the prevention of cardiac arrest. Theoretically, using pacing to control heart rate in ischemic myocardium may have a greater degree of safety and limit further ischemic damage which can occur from uncontrolled tachycardia due to pharmacological treatment aimed at increasing heart rate.

Absolute Contraindication

An absolute contraindication to the use of transcutaneous cardiac pacing has been severe hypothermia with associated bradycardia. Anecdotal reports of induction of ventricular fibrillation seemed to confirm the fear that pacing the sensitized myocardium may result in refractory ventricular fibrillation. A recent experimental animal study reported the safe and efficacious use of transcutaneous pacing as an adjunctive therapy for hypothermia induced severe bradycardia.[25] They reported no incidence of ventricular dysrhythmias induced by transcutaneous pacing. I believe cardiac pacing in profound hypothermia remains relatively contraindicated.

The primary treatment of hypothermia is rewarming, but if pacing is to be used, perhaps transcutaneous pacing may be a safer alternative than invasive pacing modalities.

Cardiac Arrests

Traditionally, asynchronous pacing has been advocated for cardiac arrests. Synchronous pacing is used when patients have some intrinsic rhythm but are hemodynamically compromised. Indications for pacing bradycardic rhythms include ineffective cardiac output evidenced by shock, altered cerebral perfusion, myocardial ischemia, premature ventricular contractions, and congestive heart failure.

Some of the pacing systems are not designed to provide asynchronous pacing. This makes their use in cardiac arrest more difficult as these machines often recognize the electrical impulse generated by a manual cardiac compression as an electrical beat. This inhibits the system and prevents a pacing electrical impulse from being delivered. These machines can be converted to asynchronous systems by removing their sensing electrodes. This also eliminates the use of the machine's monitor and an alternative ECG monitoring system must be used. Some of the machines are designed to provide both asynchronous and synchronous pacing. When using these machines during cardiopulmonary resuscitation (CPR) in a cardiac arrest, the asynchronous mode should be used. CPR causes some pulses and the operator should be careful to establish that pulses reflect the underlying rate of the pacer and not those from CPR. Additionally, the pacing often masks underlying intrinsic rhythm changes in these patients. Most commonly, ventricular fibrillation is masked. This rhythm should be treated with defibrillation and not pacing. Pacing is ineffective and, therefore, contraindicated in ventricular fibrillation. When pacing does not result in effective mechanical capture and restoration of cardiac output, the pacer should be intermittently turned "off" to assess the patient's underlying intrinsic rhythm.

Interpretation of Electrical Capture

The large wide pulse generated by transcutaneous pacemakers makes the interpretation of electrical capture more difficult. The pacemakers are designed to provide better electrocardiographic images by masking the pulse. When using standard monitors, their sensitivity should be turned down to the lowest possible setting. Electrical capture is established by the widening of the QRS complex beyond the pulse width of the pacing impulse, loss of any underlying intrinsic rhythm, and the appearance of a T wave after each pacing impulse.

If electrical capture is unsuccessful, first attempt to decrease the impedance by applying pressure to the anterior electrode. If this is unsuccessful, try to reposition the electrodes. Ideally, the initial location and configuration is over the point of maximal impulse and the scapula. Moving the anterior or posterior electrode may help provide capture. Positioning the electrodes in a V_1-V_6 standard defibrillation configuration may also be effective. Finally, some investigators have reported success in reversing the positive and negative electrodes so that the impulse goes back to front.

Pacing Failures

Some investigators have reported difficulty with transcutaneous pacing in patients having pericardial tamponade, severe chronic obstructive pulmonary disease with large impedances from hyperexpanded lung, or with excessively obese patients. In these instances, invasive cardiac pacing may prove effective. If transcutaneous pacing does not provide electrical capture, then invasive pacing techniques may prove successful in some patients. If electrical capture is obtained, but mechanical capture is not established by the development of effective cardiac output, treat the patient as if he had electromechanical dissociation.

Asystole

The prognosis for asystole remains dismal.[7,26-32] This may be true because asystole is frequently a terminal event and not the initial event in most cardiac arrests. Success in the 1950s with cardiac pacing during periods of asystole may be due to the higher incidence of short periods of asystole as a primary rhythm disturbance. Today, pharmacological treatments and permanent pacing systems have undoubtedly reduced the incidence of asystole as a primary event. It is much more common to see asystole as a terminal dysrhythmia.

Prehospital Pacing

Prehospital use of transcutaneous pacing provided an attempt at using pacing earlier in a cardiac arrest. Success has been limited with the majority of clinical trials finding no statistically different resuscitation rates for asystole. Some bradycardic arrests have been successfully paced with full neurological recovery when used early in the cardiac arrest. Clinical trials have shown either no or a small statistically significant improvement in long-term recovery.[26-32] Routine use in asystole is not advocated. Use in bradycardia may be of benefit but this has not been satisfactorily demonstrated. The introduction of combined defibrillator-pacers has allowed the prehospital personnel to use the technique earlier and minimized the equipment necessary to bring to a patient. This has resulted in wider application. The Emergency Medical System (EMS) personnel have less weight, expense, and difficulty in providing this therapy with these systems.

Pacing After Defibrillation

Dr. Jaggarao[9] investigated the use of transcutaneous pacing in conjunction with initial defibrillation for prehospital resuscitation of cardiac arrests. When patients were found in ventricular fibrillation, they were defibrillated and subsequently paced to restore a normal rhythm. He reported a significantly higher than expected success rate. The use of transcutaneous pacing to restore an effective rhythm after defibrillation has not been adequately evaluated. The possibility that transcutaneous pacing may be used to improve resuscitation after successful defibrillation should be investigated.

Pediatric Cardiac Arrests

Pediatric cardiac arrests represent a selected area of resuscitation with a larger proportion of infants having bradycardic dysrhythmias or asystole as a malignant rhythm. These patients have a much higher incidence of respiratory mechanisms for arrest, and restoration of adequate ventilation and oxygenation should be the initial treatment priority. Frequently, restoration of ventilation and oxygenation alone will result in an improved rhythm and cardiac output. When the bradycardia is persistent, the use of atropine or pacing may provide therapeutic benefit. Several studies have demonstrated the efficacy of transcutaneous pacing in providing electrical and mechanical capture in this population. Long-term survivors with intact neurological recovery are few. Some resuscitations have resulted in patients with restored hemodynamics but without neurological function. Some of these patients have become organ donors. Without cardiac pacing, this opportunity to salvage organs would have been impossible. The optimal electrode and pacing energy for infants is unknown. Commercial machines have not been designed for this use, but have been used effectively by some physicians.

Implanted Pacemaker Failures

When implanted permanent pacemakers fail and the patient's underlying rhythm results in hemodynamic compromise or cardiac arrest, transcutaneous pacing may be used to temporarily restore a regular rhythm. Use of the lowest possible energies should be attempted since conduction of the electrical impulse will occur preferentially along the existing electrode. Effective capture should be achieved at the lowest settings possible until a replacement permanent pacemaker or a transvenous pacemaker can be provided. Large electrical pulses might result in myocardial injury at the electrode site and should be avoided when possible.

Technical Considerations

The pacemakers are designed to render similar pulse widths and energies. Electrode pads are not interchangeable and each system is designed to use a particular electrode pad with its specialized impedances. Commercial machines are not designed to operate at high rates to provide override pacing capability. Some manufacturers and researchers have had their pacemakers modified to provide high rates or bursts of high rates. Square wave pulses were used by researchers establishing safety and efficacy. Many manufacturers use waveforms which are modifications of square wave, or use unique waveforms in their products. Most experimental and clinical work has been on the square wave form and the difference in wave forms have been incompletely explored. Some systems have developed a high impedance electrode which provides a more uniform electrical current delivered at the electrode interface. This may result in the ability to capture at lower energies with less muscle contraction and pain. Studies on pain have not demonstrated differences so substantial as to advocate one pacing system over the other.[19,33] My experience has been that patients resuscitated with transcutaneous pacing can be effectively treated with small doses of morphine or valium. Follow-up with these patients suggests that most do not remember pacing or the resuscitation.

Pacing during CPR

The use of transcutaneous pacing during CPR is safe to the patient and health care providers. The risk of shock is minimal and results in mild tingling if it should occur. Determining effective mechanical capture during CPR requires the operator to confirm pulses with the pacing pulses. Some models of transcutaneous pacers cannot work effectively during CPR because they are not designed to operate in the asynchronous mode. These models can be used to pace asynchronously if the electrodes to their monitor are disconnected. Other units are used in asynchronous or synchronous modalities. With these machines, asynchronous pacing is used during cardiac arrest and the synchronized pacing is used when complexes are present.

The combination of a transcutaneous pacer with a defibrillator allows the operator to use either modality. This interchangeability makes use easier, faster, more cost effective, provides less equipment weight and bulk, and generally makes the technology more available to more health care personnel. Transcutaneous pacing can be safely performed by paramedics, nurses, and most physicians. This permits the capability to provide pacing to more patients in more situations than invasive pacing systems.

Cost

The cost of transcutaneous pacing is less than for invasive pacing modalities, but it is not inconsequential. The largest equipment cost is the cumulative cost of the nonreusable, disposable electrodes. The cost of the pacemaker, or the incremental cost when combined with a defibrillator, is modest when allocated to all of the patients over the pacemaker's lifetime. One of the larger indirect costs is the required training necessary for its use. Adequate cost-benefit analysis for providing this capability to various levels of the health care system have not been performed. The apparently limited impact on long-term survival suggests that a careful outcome analysis and cost-benefit projection should be performed for various sections of the health care delivery system before it is adopted as a standard of care at all levels.

Conclusion

My use of transcutaneous pacing has evolved with time and experience. I believe it is an effective temporary pacing system. If prolonged pacing is anticipated, a transvenous pacemaker should be placed after the patient is stabilized. Transcutaneous pacing has replaced the invasive cardiac pacing systems I formerly used in cardiac arrests. I use transcutaneous pacing as an initial treatment for bradycardic cardiac arrests. I am now using it more often as an alternative to invasive pacing in prearrest rhythms or high risk rhythms in patients who may be thrombolytic candidates. I believe prevention of cardiac arrest is much more likely to be effective than treating a patient who deteriorates to the point of cardiac arrest.

The usefulness of transcutaneous cardiac pacing in cardiac arrest is limited. Successful resuscitation is unlikely unless used within the first few minutes of onset of cardiac arrest. Even under optimal circumstances, transcutaneous pacing may improve outcome in a small number of patients. Pacing in cardiac arrest may be of benefit in severe bradydysrhythmias and is unlikely to be successful in asystole. Prevention of cardiac arrest by pacing premalignant rhythms early may be the best application of this technology. As in many things, "an ounce of prevention is worth a pound of cure." (B. Franklin).

References

1. Zoll PM: Resuscitation of the heart in ventricular standstill by external electrical stimulation. N Engl J Med 247:768, 1952.
2. Zoll PM, Linenthal AJ, Norman LR, et al.: Treatment of Stokes-Adams disease by external stimulation of the heart. Circulation 9:482, 1954.
3. Zoll PM, Linenthal AJ, Norman LR: Treatment of unexpected cardiac arrest by external electric stimulation of the heart. N Engl J Med 24:68, 1956.
4. Leatham A, Cook P, Davis JG: External electric stimulator for treatment of ventricular standstill. Lancet 2:1185, 1956.
5. Falk RH, Zoll PM, Zoll RH: Safety and efficacy of noninvasive cardiac pacing : A preliminary report. N Engl J Med 309:1166, 1983.
6. Falk RH, Jacobs L, Sinclair A, et al.: External noninvasive cardiac pacing in an out-of-hospital cardiac arrest. Crit Care Med 11:779, 1983.
7. Dalsey WC, Syverud SA, Hedges JR: Emergency department use of transcutaneous cardiac pacing for cardiac arrests. Crit Care Med 13:399, 1985.
8. Zoll PM, Zoll RH, Belgard AH: External noninvasive electric stimulation of the heart. Crit Care Med 9:393, 1985.
9. Jaggarao NSV, Grainger R, Heber M, et al.: Use of automated external defibrillator-pacemaker by ambulance staff. Lancet 2:73, 1982.
10. Dalsey WC, Syverud SA, Trott A: Transcutaneous cardiac pacing. J Emerg Med 1:201, 1984.
11. Jones M, Geddes LA: Strength duration curves for cardiac pacemaking and ventricular fibrillation. Cardiovasc Res Bull 15:101, 1977.

12. Vargherse PJ, Bren G, Ross A: Electrophysiology of external cardiac pacing: A comparison study with endocardial pacing. Circulation 66:349, 1982.
13. Hedges JR, Syverud SA, Dalsey WC: Developments in transcutaneous and transthoracic pacing during bradyasystolic arrest. Ann Emerg Med 13:822, 1984.
14. Dalsey WC, Syverud SA, Hedges JR: Emergency department use of transcutaneous pacing for cardiac arrests. Crit Care Med 13:399, 1985.
15. Knowlton AA, Falk RH: External cardiac pacing during in-hospital cardiac arrest. Amer J Cardiol 57:1295, 1986.
16. Roberts JR, Greenberg MI, Crissanti J: Successful use of emergency transthoracic pacing in bradyasystolic cardiac arrest. Ann Emerg Med 13:277, 1984.
17. Syverud SA, Dalsey WC, Hedges JR: Transcutaneous and transvenous cardiac pacing for early bradyasystolic cardiac arrests. Ann Emerg Med 14:121, 1986.
18. White JM, Nowak RM, Martin GB, et al.: Immediate emergency department external cardiac pacing for prehospital bradyasystolic cardiac arrest. Ann Emerg Med 14:298, 1985.
19. Zoll PM, Zoll RH, Falk RH, et al.: External noninvasive temporary cardiac pacing: Clinical trials. Circulation 71:937, 1985.
20. Hedges JR, Syverud SA, Dalsey WC, et al.: Threshold, enzymatic, and pathologic changes associated with prolonged transcutaneous pacing in a chronic heart block model. J Emerg Med 7:1, 1989.
21. Klicklighter EJ, Syverud SA, Dalsey WC, et al.: Pathologic aspects of transcutaneous cardiac pacing. Am J Emerg Med 3:108, 1985.
22. Syverud SA, Dalsey WC, Hedges JR, et al.: Transcutaneous cardiac pacing: Determination of myocardial injury in a canine model. Ann Emerg Med 12:745, 1983.
23. Nieman JT, Rosborough JP, Garner D, et al.: External noninvasive cardiac pacing: A comparative study of two techniques with conventional endocardial pacing. PACE 7:230, 1984.
24. Syverud SA, Hedges JR, Dalsey WC, et al.: Hemodynamics of transcutaneous cardiac pacing. Am J Emerg Med 4:17, 1986.
25. Lombrino D, Dixon R, Rusnak R, et al.: Transcutaneous pacing in a hypothermic dog model. Ann Emerg Med 20:459, 1991.
26. Eitel DR, Guzzardi LJ, Stein SE, et al.: Noninvasive transcutaneous cardiac pacing in prehospital cardiac arrest. Ann Emerg Med 16:531, 1987.
27. Hedges JR, Syverud SA, Dalsey WC, et al.: Prehospital trial of emergent transcutaneous pacing. Circulation 76:1337, 1987.
28. Barthell E, Troiano P, Olson D, et al.: Prehospital external cardiac pacing: A prospective, controlled clinical trial. Ann Emerg Med 17:1221, 1988.
29. O'Toole KS, Paris PM, Heller MB, et al.: Emergency transcutaneous pacing in the management of patients with bradyasystolic rhythms. J Emerg Med 5:267, 1987.
30. Paris PM, Stewart RD, Kaplan RM, et al.: Transcutaneous pacing for

bradyasystolic cardiac arrests in prehospital care. Ann Emerg Med 14:320, 1985.
31. Cummins RO, Graves JR, Larsen MP, et al.: Prehospital transcutaneous pacing of significant bradycardias by paramedics: Clinical and system effectiveness. Prehospital Disaster Med 4:70, 1989.
32. Hedges JR, Feero S, Shultz B, et al.: Prehospital transcutaneous cardiac pacing for symptomatic bradycardia. PACE 14:1473, 1991.
33. Heller MB, Kaplan RM, Peterson J, et al.: Comparison of performance for five transcutaneous pacing devices (Abstr) Ann Emerg Med 16:493, 1987.

Chapter 6

Emergency Prehospital Transcutaneous Pacing

Jerris R. Hedges, MD, MS, FACEP

Patients who suffer a cardiac event in the prehospital setting or the emergency department are potentially salvageable. Although patients who arrest with ventricular tachycardia or fibrillation are most amenable to resuscitation, there has been hope that the other 50% of patients with cardiac events could be salvaged. The rapid provision of transcutaneous cardiac pacing has been suggested as one means to treat symptomatic bradycardia or asystolic patients with a viable myocardium. The successful application of such an intervention is dependent upon a viable myocardium,[1] a responsive and well-trained system of rescuers, and the availability of effective technology.

Cardiac care outside of the hospital is performed by individuals with various levels of training in different communities and different countries. While physicians or nurses provide such care in some countries, many parts of the world use allied health care workers (paramedics) specifically trained to provide prehospital cardiac care. In general these individuals are trained in cardiac resuscitation, clinical monitoring (including evaluation of vital signs and cardiac rhythm), stabilization of hypotension and dysrrhythmias, and the mechanics of patient transport from the prehospital setting to the hospital or between hospitals. Cardiac care outside of the hospital is

---

From *Noninvasive Transcutaneous Cardiac Pacing* edited by Pierre Birkui, M.D., Jacques Trigano, M.D., and Paul Zoll, M.D., © 1993, Futura Publishing Company, Inc., Mount Kisco, NY.

often characterized by limited resources and environmental challenges. Hence, the successful use of advanced cardiac techniques in the prehospital setting is enhanced when the personnel respond quickly and the technique is effective, frequently used, and simple to implement.

Equipment used for prehospital cardiac pacing must meet certain requirements. Because the rescuers often must carry their equipment a considerable distance from their vehicle, the device must be small and lightweight. Because prehospital care is provided in extremes of temperature and lighting, and because the device may be dropped or otherwise physically abused when repeatedly moved, the instrument must be sturdy and function under a wide range of environmental conditions. Since multiple individuals will use the device on an intermittent basis, the device must be simple to use with few knobs or settings. Finally, because all prehospital and interhospital transport teams must justify equipment purchases, the device and add-on disposable equipment (e.g., pacing pads and monitoring electrodes) must be reasonably priced.

Recently, portable battery operated stand-alone transcutaneous pacemakers and combination pacemaker-defibrillator devices have been developed for prehospital use. Many of these devices have been clinically evaluated in the prehospital setting. Through these investigations, we have begun to determine the role of transcutaneous cardiac pacing for prehospital cardiac patients. This chapter will review clinical experience relevant to the emergency department and prehospital setting, the indications and contraindications for transcutaneous pacing in the prehospital setting, clinical use of the devices, and complications with device use. The use of transcutaneous pacing in emergency departments is guided by the same principles although equipment specifications are less demanding.

Historical Background

Early emergency department studies of transcutaneous pacing using modern equipment verified that electrical and mechanical capture were more likely with transcutaneous pacing than transvenous pacing in the setting of low blood flow.[2] Emergency department and in-hospital series found that long-term survival occurred primarily in the setting of transcutaneous pacing within ten minutes of hemodynamic collapse.[3-5]

Prehospital reports of transcutaneous pacing have largely been case series of pacing used for patients with collapse due to bradycardia or asystole. The earliest report using a modern era pacemaker by Jaggarao et al. described a combination pacemaker-defibrillator used for selected patients including postdefibrillation bradycardia patients.[6] Subsequent series described the use of the device to resuscitate patients with bradycardias which failed isoproterenol and atropine therapy, pulseless bradycardias (mainly, idioventricular rhythms), and asystole.[7-10] These studies were characterized by a long duration from collapse until pacing and a lack of controls. Of note is the consistent reporting of dismal outcomes with asystolic and pulseless bradycardia patients. One prehospital system reported no long-term survivors out of 19 pulseless individuals (13 asystolic and 6 bradycardic) who were paced within 10 minutes of a witnessed collapse.[10]

Two controlled prehospital studies similarly noted a poor outcome for these patients.[11,12] Unfortunately, there was considerable delay in the initiation of pacing for the majority of these patients as well. However, the patients in the trial by Barthell et al.[12] who presented with a pulse and developed hemodynamically significant bradycardia fared significantly better than those patients treated with atropine alone. Additional case series of favorable outcomes in patients with hemodynamically significant bradycardia have been reported from different prehospital care systems.[13-15] One series is from a system that had previously reported that patients paced after failing drug therapy universally also failed pacing.[8-13] This observation raises the question as to whether earlier use of pacing would have saved many of their patients from the earlier series. Two other prehospital systems[14,15] and one transport program[16] have reported case series which suggest that NTCP can salvage bradycardia patients who present with a pulse but who fail atropine therapy.

In a review of patients with hemodynamically significant bradycardia from Thurston County, Washington, USA, my colleagues and I obtained similar results (unpublished data; Fig. 1). Of 51 bradycardia patients with witnessed cardiovascular decompensation, 27 (53%) were paced. There were no significant differences between the paced patients and those without pacing for mean times from collapse until cardiopulmonary resuscitation, paramedic arrival, and a paceable rhythm or from paramedic arrival until a paceable rhythm. Overall, emergency department arrival with a palpable pulse (26% vs

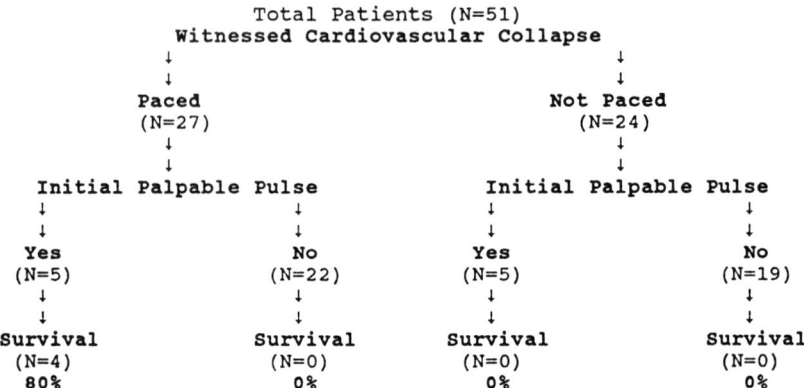

Figure 1. *Outcome of prehospital patients with symptomatic bradycardia. Thurston County, Washington, USA.*

13%, p = 0.20) and survival to hospital discharge (15% vs 0%, p = 0.07) tended to be better for the paced group. Only in the paced group was the presence of a palpable pulse upon paramedic arrival associated with survival to hospital discharge (80% vs 0%, p = 0.004). Comparison of survival to hospital discharge for paced and nonpaced patients with a palpable pulse upon paramedic arrival showed a significantly better survival for those who were paced (80% vs 0%, p = 0.024). Hence, prehospital transcutaneous cardiac pacing appears to be most beneficial in those patients with bradycardia who have a palpable pulse when first seen.

In summary, emergency department and prehospital studies support the premise that clinical response to transcutaneous cardiac pacing is dependent upon viable myocardium.[1] The patient with little functional myocardium is unlikely to benefit from pacing. Similarly, the longer the period of ischemia, the less likely the patient will be to benefit from pacing. Hence, if transcutaneous pacing is to be successful in the prehospital setting, the prehospital rescuers must be notified immediately of a patient at risk for a cardiac event and arrive promptly at the patient's side; the team must be equipped with a reliable pacemaker device with which they are familiar and which they can rapidly implement; they must recognize the low flow state associated with perfusing bradycardias and promptly initiate transcutaneous cardiac pacing; and the device used must be well-tolerated by the patient until the need has passed or transvenous cardiac pacing can be instituted.

Indications

The transcutaneous pacemaker is indicated as either a standby device for patients at risk for symptomatic bradycardia or for the therapy of symptomatic bradycardia (Fig. 2). Patients who would benefit from a pacemaker as a standby device are those suspected of or proven to have had cardiac syncope, heart block, implanted pacemaker dysfunction, myocardial infarction with conduction defects, hyperkalemia, beta-agonist[17] or cardiac glycoside intoxication,[18], or similar conditions which may be associated with bradycardia development.

A condition recently added to this category is the standby use of transcutaneous pacing for patients receiving thrombolytic therapy for myocardial infarction and at risk for infarct-related or postreperfusion

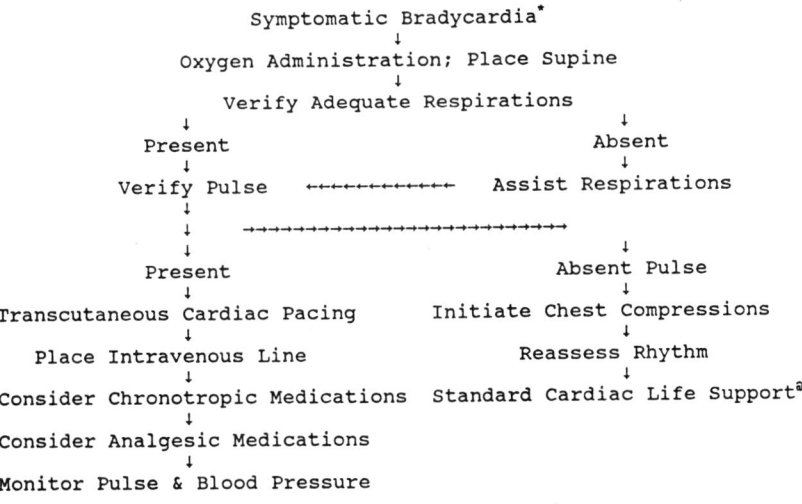

Figure 2. *Prehospital resuscitation algorithm incorporating use of transcutaneous cardiac pacing. *See text for examples. Prehospital NTCP is not indicated for asystole unless collapse is witnessed, cardiopulmonary resuscitation is immediate, and pacing is initiated within 10 minutes of collapse. @ Standard advanced cardiac life support should follow protocols for specific cardiac rhythm. While NTCP is unlikely to benefit this group of patients, pacing is warranted if the patient develops a pulse with ventilation, chest compression, and medications.*

bradycardia. Transvenous pacing is generally contraindicated in this setting because of the potential for hemorrhage with catheter sheath placement and catheter passage. While few prehospital systems are administering thrombolytic agents outside of the hospital, many prehospital systems are transporting patients who have been given these agents in an emergency department prior to transport to a cardiac center. Similarly, many emergency departments are administering these agents. Hence, a transcutaneous pacing device for standby use is considered an essential piece of equipment for these emergency departments and prehospital systems.

Patients with symptomatic bradycardia may present with lightheadedness, confusion, dyspnea, chest pain, and peripheral vasoconstriction. These patients may tolerate the bradycardia for long durations if kept supine and administered fluids and oxygen. However more commonly, these patients suffer cardiac arrest within minutes if not promptly treated. Traditional management has included therapy with atropine and beta-agonist agents (e.g., isoproterenol or dopamine). These agents are not without complications. Commonly their use is either without effect upon cardiac rate, of a brief duration, or associated with marked tachycardia which can potentially produce further ischemia from an increased myocardial demand. Transcutaneous pacing is more appropriate for these patients since it bypasses the diseased conducting system and ensures a fixed rate response.

As noted above, transcutaneous pacing appears to have little benefit for the patient with asystole or a pulseless bradycardia. Although some patients with a viable myocardium who sustain a cardiac arrest and are promptly paced from a bradycardic rhythm are expected to benefit, patients with bradycardia or asystole and without a pulse for more than ten minutes do not appear to benefit from pacing. The role of transcutaneous pacing for postdefibrillation asystole or bradycardia is unknown. Although clinical survivors with transcutaneous pacing have been noted for this category, the role of pacing is uncertain. Animal studies and clinical series have not supported transcutaneous pacing for this condition.[11,19,20]

Contraindications

Little attention has been paid to potential contraindications to transcutaneous pacing. Dalsey et al.[2] report that one of their patients who was hypothermic developed ventricular fibrillation when paced for a symptomatic bradycardia. They recommended that pacing be avoided for this group of patients until further study can be done. Theoretically, the known irritability of the cold myocardium supports this concept.

Certain patients will find transcutaneous pacing to be intolerable as a result of skeletal muscle contraction and painful skin receptor stimulation.[21] The presence of severe pain upon pacing represents a relative contraindication to transcutaneous pacing. The rescuer has several options in this situation. The patient can be sedated and provided analgesia (some investigators have used nitrous oxide,[22] while others have used narcotics and benzodiazepine agents). Alternatively, the clinician can use the pacemaker in a standby mode if the patient is able clinically to tolerate the bradycardia when placed in a supine position and administered supplemental oxygen. When there is evidence of poor perfusion without transcutaneous pacing, I prefer to provide pacing and analgesia until transvenous pacing can be undertaken.

Equipment

A variety of transcutaneous pacing devices have been manufactured. Recent legal claims of patent infringement have reduced the number of products on the market. Since this is a dynamic area, this chapter will only review the features which are desirable for these devices. Comparison of different commercial products is provided elsewhere.[22,23] As noted in the introduction, the devices must be small, lightweight, durable, reliable, simple to operate, and relatively inexpensive.

Since devices which are used on a daily basis and consistently taken to the patient as a piece of standard equipment are more likely to be used efficiently, pacemaker-defibrillator devices are more desirable in the prehospital setting than stand-alone pacemaker devices which generally function as supplemental equipment. Combination pacemaker-defibrillator units also are advantageous in that the same monitor can be used for visual rhythm and pacemaker capture confirmation. The least expensive stand-alone pacemakers do not come with a monitor and hence capture is determined by clinical evaluation (alertness or palpation of a pulse). Because skeletal contraction occurs with external thoracic stimulation, it is often difficult to determine when a pulse is present. Furthermore, the device must be periodically turned "off" during resuscitation when a pulse is questionable to determine if ventricular fibrillation has occurred.

Each device needs a low battery indicator and preferably should contain a backup battery or the capability of functioning "off" of a standard electrical power cable during battery recharging. Because prolonged pacing during long transports may be required, these devices must have a battery capacity permitting pacing for a minimum of one hour if used during patient transportation.

Pacing pads are generally designed for use with one pacemaker device. Although the pads may be interchanged on some units, the performance varies considerably.[25] The resultant impedance change may result in a more painful pacing experience for awake patients or may result in inability to capture altogether. Sufficient stock of the appropriate pacing pads must be kept by the prehospital system to optimize pacing benefit.

Clinical Use

When used in the prehospital setting or the emergency department as a standby pacing mechanism, the electrode pads should be placed according to each manufacturer's instructions. Generally a cathode (negative) electrode pad is placed over the site of the apical impulse of the heart. The placement of the posterior pad is less critical, but commonly located on the posterior thorax to the left of the spine directly behind the anterior pad.[26] Obviously the opposite (right hemithorax) would be used for anterior pad placement in the setting of dextrocardia.

Monitoring leads and electrode pads are attached to the pacing generator. If the pacing generator has a monitor, the underlying rhythm is monitored on the pacing generator monitor. If the device has sensing capability, one can test the sensing function by turning the current to a low setting and the rate to a setting greater than the patient's intrinsic rate. The patient's intrinsic beats should be sensed with pacing performed only between intrinsic beats. It is wise to determine the patient's threshold to pacing as well. With the rate set above the patient's intrinsic rate, the current output is increased until capture occurs on the monitor. The patient should be forewarned of the expected discomfort and the device turned "off" once capture has been confirmed. If there is a high risk of bradycardia, the device is placed in the demand mode, the desired pacing rate set, the current adjusted to a level just above threshold, and appropriate analgesia and sedation provided. When the need for pacing is less likely, the device parameters may be set, but the device kept in the monitor mode only. Should bradycardia occur, the device is then turned "on" to the demand mode and appropriate analgesia and sedation administered. When there is no demand mode on the pacemaker, visual monitoring with manual institution of pacing at the preestablished settings is used when bradycardia develops. When the device has no intrinsic monitor, the monitor leads should go to a separate cardiac monitor (e.g., defibrillator device monitor). Some pacing devices also have a filter to permit damping of pacing complexes with observance of capture on the defibrillator monitor when the pacemaker is turned "on." Otherwise the pacemaker spikes will dominate the monitor when the device is activated.

When the patient is hemodynamically unstable, the pacing device should be set to a rate of 80–100 ppm and the maximum device output used to obtain immediate capture. The output is decreased to a level just above threshold by trial and error. While complexes can be monitored for capture in those devices with a built-in monitor or electrical filter (as described above), the best measure of clinical effect is monitoring of femoral pulses or peripheral blood pressure using palpation or preferably a Doppler flow device. When the patient becomes more alert with pacing, careful assessment must be performed to determine if the improvement in alertness is related to improved perfusion or to increased pain from electrical stimulation of the thorax. Analgesia and sedation are useful in this setting to permit careful assessment of perfusion. Pulse oxymetry may also be helpful in this setting in that only when perfusion is adequate will the pulse oximeter device provide a satisfactory reading.[27] If the patient is intubated, carbon dioxide elimination as detected by an electronic CO_2 meter or disposable membrane CO_2 detector (e.g., FEF End-Tidal CO_2 detector, Fenem, Inc) may also be useful guides to perfusion.[28] Only with satisfactory perfusion of the lungs will adequate CO_2 elimination occur.

The benefit from transcutaneous pacing is expected to be greatest when the technique is initiated as a high priority during resuscitation. Transcutaneous pacing for the symptomatic bradycardia patient should only follow oxygenation, ventilation, and cardiac massage (when indicated) in the resuscitation sequence. Supplemental volume and drug therapy should follow rather than precede pacing efforts.

The presence of a pericardial effusion or tension pneumothorax will raise the energy requirements for pacing.[29] In general, patients who are found pulseless in the prehospital setting with a paceable rhythm rarely respond to pacing. Furthermore, the value of pacing postcardioversion or postdefibrillation rhythms is unknown. Transcutaneous pacing should be reserved for those patients needing hemodynamic support or who have suffered a cardiac arrest within ten minutes of pacing availability, assuming that cardiopulmonary resuscitation was promptly instituted.

Complications

Activation of the pacemaker device before proper application of the electrode to the skin or failing to inactivate the device when removing an electrode can lead to a mild electrical shock when the rescuer contacts the electrode conducing surface. While startling, there is no significant harm from such contact. Commercial electrodes, if properly applied, have sufficient insulation on the posterior surface that manual chest compressions can be performed during resuscitation while the device is pacing the heart without threat of rescuer shock.

Patient injury from transcutaneous cardiac pacing is unlikely with current devices and electrodes. One case of a cutaneous burn occurred in an infant who was paced for an extended period of time (nearly two days) without movement of the electrodes.[30] While anatomical animal studies[29,31] have shown minimal myocardial microscopic damage with prolonged pacing, physiological studies suggest these findings are of no clinical significance,[29,32] and clinical studies have also failed to identify significant myocardial injury.[33]

Of greater importance is when the device is used and myocardial capture does not occur. The rescuer must verify the electrode placement and ensure that tight contact with the skin occurs, be certain that all leads are attached, determine that the battery is charged or the device is functioning while plugged into an electrical outlet, and ensure that all device settings are appropriate. Maximum energy should be used when the patient is markedly hypotensive or pulseless until better perfusion is assured.

Because the output of the device is considerably greater than the standard transvenous pacemaker generator, the pacemaker spike may produce monitor artefact and stimulate electrical capture unless the pacer spike is appropriately damped. One may have difficulty noticing that ventricular fibrillation has occurred and that defibrillation rather than pacing should be instituted. Hence, close clinical monitoring of the patient response with brief, occasional periods of electrical monitoring while the pacemaker device is "off" is necessary when a second monitor device is used.

Some earlier versions of the pacemaker device had no low battery warning or the device could not be operated while the battery was recharging. The rescuer must be aware of these design limitations and take appropriate actions (e.g., carry a spare charged battery) should devices with these design characteristics be used.

The existence of different devices in the same institution also raises an interesting dilemma. At times pacemaker-dependent patients must be changed from one device to another when the electrode pads for the two devices are not interchangeable. The two medical teams must be aware of potential compatibility problems and work quickly to convert a patient from one device to another. The general process for changing devices is as follows. While pacing the patient with the first device, the second device should be preset to the settings currently in use with the first device. Preferably the current setting is set slightly higher than for the first device to ensure capture; it can be decreased subsequently. With all pads attached to their respective devices, the first device is quickly turned "off" and the electrodes removed. The electrodes for the second unit are then attached and the device turned "on" immediately.

Conclusions

While half of out-of-hospital cardiac arrests involve bradycardia or asystolic rhythms and many patients with ventricular fibrillation develop a paceable rhythm postdefibrillation, few of these patients will benefit from transcutaneous cardiac pacing. The modality appears most useful for patients with some perfusion in the setting of bradycardia and hemodynamic compromise. Case series and controlled prehospital studies suggest that this modality is of significant benefit for patients with a potentially life-threatening bradycardia. Prehospital systems with rapid response times, prolonged transport times, and a high percentage of cardiac patients are most likely to benefit from the availability of this technique. Similar factors apply to the use of transcutaneous pacing in the emergency department, although many equipment design features important for prehospital use are less important for pacing in the emergency department.

References

1. Hedges JR, Syverud SA, Dalsey WC, et al.: Developments in transcutaneous and transthoracic pacing during bradyasystolic arrest. Ann Emerg Med 13:822, 1984.
2. Dalsey WC, Syverud SA, Hedges JR: Emergency department use of transcutaneous pacing for cardiac arrests. Crit Care Med 13:399, 1985.
3. Clinton JE, Zoll PM, Zoll RH, et al.: Emergency noninvasive external cardiac pacing. J Emerg Med 2:155, 1985.
4. Zoll PM, Zoll RH, Falk RH, et al.: External noninvasive temporary cardiac pacing: Clinical trials. Circulation 71:937, 1985.
5. Syverud SA, Dalsey WC, Hedges JR: Transcutaneous and transvenous cardiac pacing for early bradyasystolic cardiac arrest. Ann Emerg Med 15:121, 1986.
6. Jaggarao NSV, Grainger R, Heber M, et al.: Use of automated external defibrillator-pacemaker by ambulance staff. Lancet 2:73, 1982.
7. Falk RH, Jacobs L, Sinclair A, et al.: External noninvasive cardiac pacing in an out-of-hospital cardiac arrest. Crit Care Med 11:779, 1983.
8. Paris PM, Stewart RD, Kaplan R, et al.: Transcutaneous pacing for bradyasystolic cardiac arrests in prehospital care. Ann Emerg Med 14:320, 1985.
9. Eitel DR, Guzzardi LR, Stein SE, et al.: Noninvasive transcutaneous cardiac pacing in prehospital cardiac arrest. Ann Emerg Med 16:531, 1987.
10. Vukov LF, White RD: Emergency transcutaneous pacemakers in prehospital cardiac arrest (letter). Ann Emerg Med 17:554, 1988.
11. Hedges JR, Syverud SA, Dalsey WC, et al.: Prehospital trial of emergency transcutaneous cardiac pacing. Circulation 76:1337, 1987.
12. Barthell E, Troiano P, Olso, D, et al.: Prehospital external cardiac pacing: A prospective, controlled clinical trial. Ann Emerg Med 17:1221, 1988.
13. O'Toole KS, Paris PM, Heller MB, et al.: Emergency transcutaneous pacing in the management of patients with bradyasystolic rhythms. J Emerg Med 5:267, 1987.

14. Goldstein J, Eitel D, Cramer W, et al.: The use of prehospital external cardiac pacing in bradycardic patients (abstr). Ann Emerg Med 19:478, 1990.
15. Cummins RO, Graves JR, Larsen MP, et al.: Prehospital transcutaneous pacing of significant bradycardias by paramedics: Clinical and system effectiveness (abstr). Prehosp Disaster Med 4:70, 1989.
16. Vukov LF, Johnson DQ: External transcutaneous pacemakers in interhospital transport of cardiac patients. Ann Emerg Med 18:738, 1989.
17. Kenyon CJ. Aldinger GE, Joshipura P, et al.: Successful resuscitation using external cardiac pacing in beta adrenergic antagonist-induced bradyasystolic arrest. Ann Emerg Med 17:711, 1988.
18. Cummins RO, Haulman J, Quan L, et al.: Near-fatal yew berry intoxication treated with external cardiac pacing and digoxin-specific FAB antibody fragments. Ann Emerg Med 19:38, 1990.
19. Niemann JT, Haynes KS, Garner D, et al.: Postcountershock pulseless rhythms: Response to CPR, artificial cardiac pacing and adrenergic agonists. Ann Emerg Med 15:112, 1986.
20. Niemann JT, Adomian GE, Garner D, et al.: Endocardial and transcutaneous cardiac pacing, calcium chloride, and epinephrine in postcountershock asystole and bradycardias. Crit Care Med 13:699, 1985.
21. Heller MB, Peterson J, Ilkhanipour K, et al.: A comparative study of five transcutaneous pacing devices in unanesthetized human volunteers. Prehosp Disaster Med 4:15, 1989.
22. Kaplan RM, Heller MB, McPherson J, et al.: An evaluation of nitrous oxide analgesia during transcutaneous pacing. Prehosp Disaster Med 5:145, 1990.
23. Dillon DJ: Transcutaneous pacemakers. Health Devices 17:39, 1988.
24. Bocka JJ: External transcutaneous pacemakers. Ann Emerg Med 18:1280, 1989.
25. Kaplan RM, Heller MB, Paris PM, et al.: The effect of different combinations of external pacemaker and pads on pacing thresholds, capture rate, and patient tolerance (abstr). Ann Emerg Med 17:750, 1988.
26. Falk RH, Ngai STA: External cardiac pacing: Influence of electrode placement on pacing threshold. Crit Care Med 14:931, 1986.
27. Field DL, Hedges JR: Noninvasive assessment and delivery of oxygen and inhaled medications. In Clinical Procedures in Emergency Medicine. Roberts JR, Hedges JR (eds). Saunders WB Co, Philadelphia, 1991, p. 70.
28. Federiuk CS, Sanders AB: Artificial perfusion during cardiac arrest. In: Clinical Procedures in Emergency Medicine. Roberts JR, Hedges JR (eds). Saunders WB Co, Philadelphia, 1991, p. 234.
29. Hedges JR, Syverud SA, Dalsey WC, et al.: Threshold, enzymatic, and pathologic changes associated with prolonged transcutaneous pacing in a chronic heart block model. J Emerg Med 7:1, 1989.
30. Pride HB, McKinley DF: Third-degree burns from use of an external cardiac pacing device. Crit Care Med 18:572, 1990.
31. Kicklighter EJ, Syverud SA, Dalsey WC, et al.: Pathological aspects of transcutaneous cardiac pacing. Am J Emerg Med 3:108, 1985.

32. Syverud SA, Hedges JR, Dalsey WC, et al.: Hemodynamics of transcutaneous cardiac pacing. Am J Emerg Med 4:17, 1986.
33. Madsen K, Pedersen F, Grande P, et al.: Normal myocardial enzymes and normal echocardiographic findings during noninvasive transcutaneous pacing. PACE 11:1188, 1988.

Chapter 7

Prehospital Prospective Controlled Transcutaneous Cardiac Pacing: 24-Month Clinical Trial

Carolyn J. Kenyon, MD,
Glenn E. Aldinger, MD FACEP

We undertook a 2-year prospective controlled clinical trial of prehospital noninvasive transcutaneous cardiac pacing (NTCP) in an Advanced Life Support (ALS) paramedic system with a mean response time to the scene of 3.9±3.3 minutes to evaluate its success and practicality in this setting.

Profound bradycardia and asystole are often seen in the human cardiac arrest state, having been shown to account for from 30% to 60% of initial arrest rhythms. Survival of patients with bradyasystolic cardiac rhythms is uniformly dismal. Statistics from large studies of bradyasystolic arrest victims treated without external pacing, but under otherwise optimal conditions (in which paramedics responded in under 4 minutes to a witnessed arrest with bystander CPR in progress and followed Advanced Cardiac Life Support (ACLS) protocol), show from 0% to 12% initial "save" rates and in most studies, under 1% long-term survival to discharge from a hospital.[1-7]

Various studies have now shown a potential salvageability of

From *Noninvasive Transcutaneous Cardiac Pacing* edited by Pierre Birkui, M.D., Jacques Trigano, M.D., and Paul Zoll, M.D., © 1993, Futura Publishing Company, Inc., Mount Kisco, NY.

some bradyasystolic arrest victims with early application of NTCP.[8-24] These studies illustrate that electrical capture and pacing of the heart with return of measurable pulse and blood pressure is possible. Zoll reported 23 of 26 patients paced early survived to discharge and Madsen noted similar success for 19 of 22 acutely paced patients.[10,21] It is an often repeated hypothesis that by introducing cardiac pacing sooner in the course of a bradyasystolic arrest, that many more patients could be saved.[8,11,12,13,15]

There are numerous therapeutic modalities that have been used to increase the heart rate during cardiac arrest. The American Heart Association presently recommends atropine followed preferentially by an external transcutaneous pacemaker or isoproterenol if a pacer is not available for symptomatic bradycardiac arrhythmias. Epinephrine followed by atropine and pacing are recommended for ventricular asystole.[25]

Case reports of field success with transcutaneous pacing generated interest in the application of rapid noninvasive cardiac pacing to the prehospital setting. Several studies soon followed.[26-34] Only three of these[27,28,34] utilized some form of control population, and no study exceeded 112 paced patients. Despite earlier enthusiasm for early pacing use in the field, no numerically significant enhanced survival could be demonstrated as a result of its use. Advocates cited the case reports of successes, emphasized the delays to rapid pacing in studies to date, and called for adoption of early pacing as well as for continued study. Prehospital pacing capability became an issue for cost conscious paramedic systems under pressure to acquire state-of-the-art medical equipment.

Methods

From March 1987 through March 1989, 604 consecutive adult patients presenting in the prehospital setting with asystole, complete heart block (CHB/third degree block), pulseless idioventricular rhythms (PIVR), and symptomatic bradycardia from cardiac causes, and who did not initially respond to AHA treatment protocols, were enrolled in the study. The protocol for pacer implementation was designed to encourage and expedite its use when available. Traumatic arrests and patients under age 18 were excluded.

Upon identification of a protocol rhythm (Fig. 1), paramedics

Protocol

All Patients: American Heart Association Guidelines

    Asystole CPR
                   Establish IV
                   0.5-1.0 mg epinephrine(1:10,000)
                   1.0 mg atropine

    Bradycardia 0.5 - 1.0 mg atropine

Paced Patients:
        Rate: 80
        Mode: Demand
  Initial output: Asystole 150 mAmp
                   Bradycardia 40 mAmp

Figure 1. *Transcutaneous-pacer study protocol.*

were instructed to continue ALS treatment already in progress. If not already done, transcutaneous pacer electrode pads were applied: anterior chest pad placed in apical area, posterior chest pad placed on the back slightly left of T_4.

For asystole/PIVR, initiation of transcutaneous pacing was to begin. (Asystole was to be verified with two (2) separate leads or axis determinations). Appropriate epinephrine and atropine were administered. If asystole continued, and if a transcutaneous pacer was available, paramedics were to initiate the transcutaneous pacer protocol and begin pacing without delay and without awaiting the order of a telemetry physician. Pacer settings for asystole are: rate: 80 ppm; sensitivity: auto (demand); output: 150 mA. For symptomatic bradycardias/AV blocks, paramedics were instructed to establish telemetry contact to obtain orders for atropine, and for pacing should the patient not improve. Pacer settings for bradycardia: rate: 80 ppm; sensitivity: auto (demand); output: 40 mA with incremental increases until consistent capture was obtained. Transcutaneous pacing always continued en route to the hospital unless otherwise ordered by the telemetry physician.

Characteristics of the System

The contiguous communities covering 71.9 square miles and a population of 320,000 on the northern boundary of Chicago are served by 18 advanced life support ambulances manned by 287 EMT-P paramedics.

There are five hospitals in the service area. All paramedics were instructed and tested on use of the Pace Aid® and the study protocol immediately prior to the initiation of the study.

Equipment

A portable cardiac pacemaker, Pace Aid® Model 53 (Cardiac Resuscitator Corporation, Portland, Oregon), was used throughout the study. The pacer can operate in two modes: asynchronous and demand. Rate can be varied from 50 to 160 ppm, and current output from 10 to 150 mA. Pulse duration is uniphasic (10 msec). The pacer weighs 2.7 kg (6 pounds).

Statistical Methods

Chi-square, Fisher's exact test, one- and two-tailed t-tests, and analysis of variance were applied where appropriate with a significance level of p less than or equal to 0.05 accepted.

Systematic allocation of pacers was accomplished by rotating the 11 pacers on a monthly basis between 18 advanced life support ambulances. No individual service area was ever without at least one pacer. All nonpaced patients served as controls. Withdrawals from pacer available group occurred when either:

1. patient eligible for study and pacer available but not used;
2. patient eligible for study and pacer broken. These patients were assigned to the control category.

Withdrawals from evaluation in specific data categories occurred because of data missing on ambulance run report or Supplemental Pacer Protocol Report sheet for that category/item of data.

Informed Consent

Informed consent could not be obtained for this study. The patients were considered to be in a life-threatening situation and time was not available to explain the procedure and obtain consent from the patients' families. This situation meets the Food and Drug Administration (FDA) guidelines for investigational devices exceptions to the informed consent rule.[35]

The Institutional Review Board of Saint Francis Hospital granted approval for the study without revisions on September 10, 1986.

Results

Six hundred and fourteen adults met study criteria in the 24-month period. Ten lacked critical information and could not be included in the study. Of 228 patients with a pacer available, 145 were actually paced and the remaining 83 were evaluated with the 376 patients for whom no pacer had been available and thus served as controls. Of the 145 paced patients, 86 (59%) showed capture, 21 (14%) developed pulses, 10 (7%) were resuscitated and admitted, and 4 (3%) survived to be discharged. Of the 459 patients not paced, 57 (12%) regained pulses with standard ACLS care, 52 (11%) were admitted, and 32 (7%) were discharged (p = NS, Fig. 2).

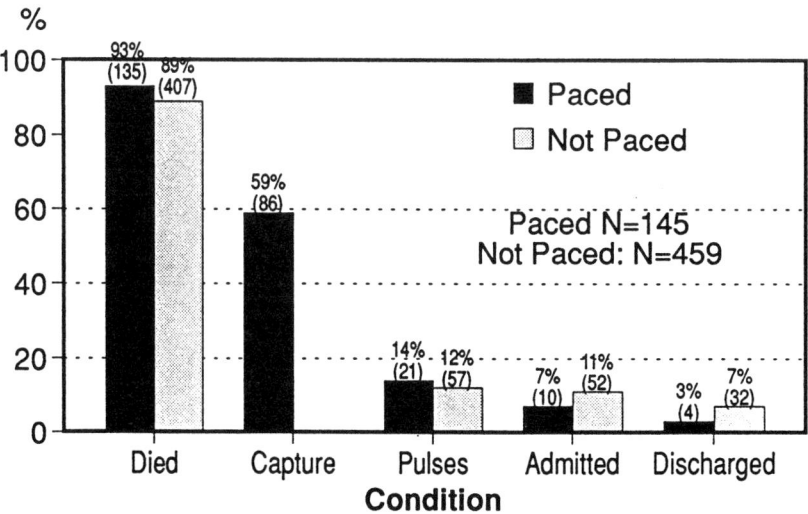

Figure 2. *Prehospital transcutaneous pacer study. Summary of the results.*

Analysis by specific rhythm subgroups showed no significant differences in resuscitation or survival rates for paced and control patients (Figs. 3, 4). All symptomatic bradycardias were evaluated. Twenty-one were paced. Of these, 16 (76.2%) died, 5 (23.8%) were admitted, and 3 (14.3%) survived to discharge. For 82 nonpaced patients, 48 (58.5%) died, 34 (41.5%) were admitted, and 22 (26.8%) survived. For 462 arrests with asystole as a treated rhythm, 118 were paced and 5 (4.3%) admitted. There were 44 that were not paced and 12 (3.5%) of these were resuscitated by standard ACLS care and admitted. Arrests where asystole was not present as the initial rhythm but rather developed later (late asystole) number 236. Of these, 3 of 58 (5.2%) paced patients and 11 of 178 (6.2%) nonpaced were admitted. No paced patients survived to discharge, but 6 (3.4%) nonpaced patients did (Fig. 5).

All cases that listed asystole as one of the treated rhythms at any point during the resuscitation were identified and removed creating a subset of nonasystole arrests. For these remaining cases, bradycardia, PIVR, and CHB were then separately evaluated. Twenty bradycardiac cases were identified. One of 3 paced, and 6 of 17 nonpaced patients survived to admission. Similarly, 31 PIVR cases revealed 1 of 7 paced and 1 of 24 controls were admitted. Of 12 CHB cases, 1 of 3 paced and 6 of 9 nonpaced were resuscitated.

All groups were comparable in terms of age, sex, witnessed events, mean time to CPR, ACLS, and scene response time (Table 1). Males comprised 56.4%, (62% of paced and 54% of controls). Mean age was 73.15 ± 14.07 years (paced: 73.9 ± 12.1, controls: 72.9 ± 14.7). Mean response time to scene from receipt of call was 3.94 ± 3.34 minutes (3.90 minutes paced, and 3.94 minutes controls). Twenty two percent had response time less than or equal to 2 minutes, 50% were under 3 minutes, 75% had response times under 4 minutes, 98% under 8 minutes, and 99% under 10 minutes.

Factors known to affect survival were compared (Table 2). For known response time from receipt of call less than or equal to 4 minutes, 8 of 104 paced patients were admitted, and 3 were discharged. Thirty four of 335 controls were resuscitated and 17 survived. In arrests with known response time greater than 4 minutes, 1 of 38 paced patients was admitted and survived while 18 of 111 controls were admitted and 15 of these lived ($p = NS$).

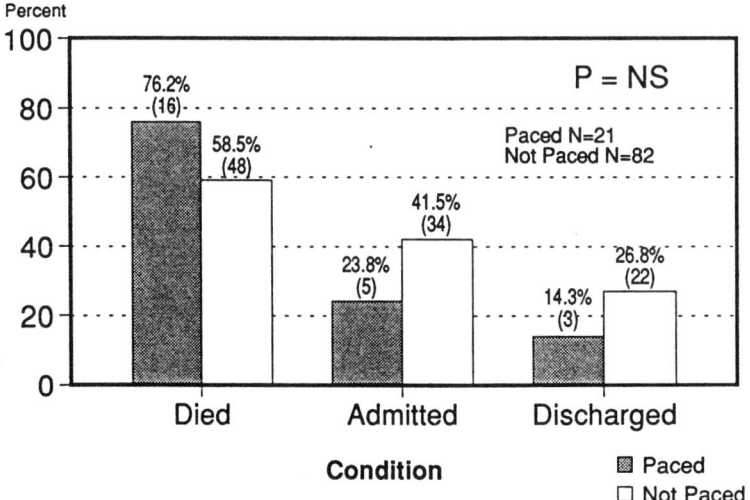

Figure 3: *All symptomatic bradycardias.*

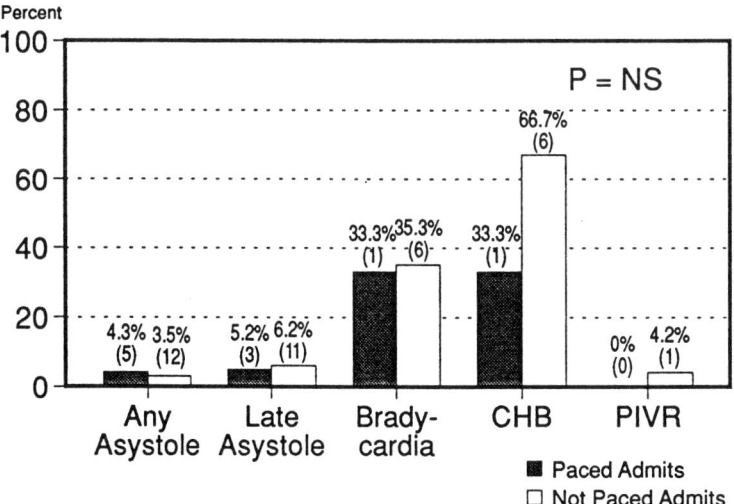

Figure 4: *Initial survival by rhythm. Arrests with any asystolic rhythm are compared to arrests with asystole witnessed by paramedics and not initially present, and to other paced rhythms that did not have any asystole present during the arrest.*

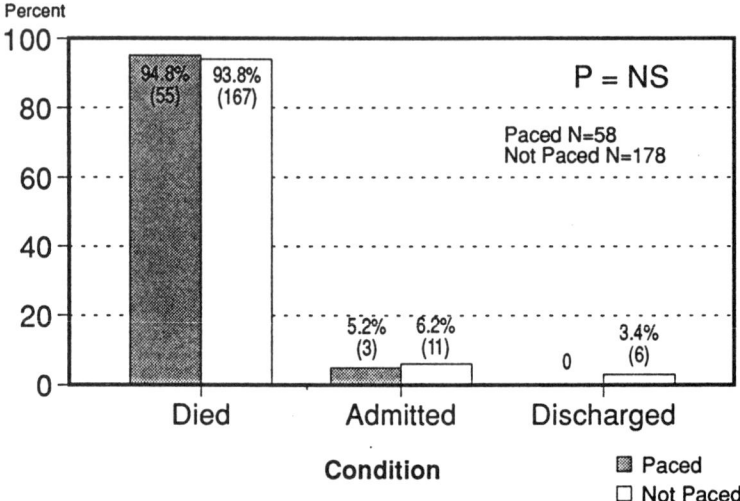

Figure 5: *Asystole later in arrest. Survival for arrests in which asystole was not present initially but developed later during the arrest.*

Table 1. Comparison of Study Group Characteristics and Variables

	Variables Paced	Not Paced	Significance
Age	73.9 ± 12.1 yr	72.9 ± 14.7 yr	NS
Sex Male	62%	54%	NS
Witnessed Arrest	26%	32%	NS
Mean Response Time	3.90 min.	3.96 min.	NS
Time to ACLS < 8 min	52.9%	44.9%	NS
Time to hospital	38.5 min.	32.0 min.	p<.0005

A total of 528 cases included witnessed vs unwitnessed information. Of these, 26% of paced and 32% of controls had witnessed events. Two of 36 (5.6%) paced patients were admitted, one was discharged. Eight of 125 (6.4%) controls were resuscitated, and 6 survived (p = NS).

Time from arrest to initiation of CPR was available for 496 cases. Thirty-three (26.2%) of paced and 132 (26.8%) of nonpaced patients had CPR within 4 minutes of arrest. An additional 50 paced (39.7%)

Table 2. Comparison of Paced and Unpaced (Control) Groups with Factors Known to Affect Survival from an Arrest

Parameter	—Paced— Total	Admitted [%]	—Not Paced— Total	Admitted [%]
Response < 4 min.	104	8 [7.7]	335	34 [10.1]
Response > 4 min.	38	1 [2.6]	111	18 [6.2]
ACLS < 8 min.	63	2 [3.2]	129	4 [13.8]
ACLS > 8 min.	56	2 [3.6]	156	2 [1.3]
Witnessed Arrest	36	2 [5.6]	125	8 [6.4]

and 146 (39.5%) nonpaced patients had CPR initiated between 4 and 12 minutes from arrest. The remaining one-third (43 paced and 125 nonpaced) were down over 12 minutes before CPR was started. Chi-square analysis showed no significant difference between groups (p = .9921). When CPR was initiated within 4 minutes, 2 (6.1%) paced and 9 (9.1%) nonpaced patients were admitted. Of those individuals who had CPR within 4 to 12 minutes, 4 (8%) paced and 5 (3.4%) nonpaced patients were admitted. When CPR was started more than 12 minutes after the start of an arrest, none of the paced patients and 2 (1.6%) nonpaced patients survived to be admitted. Of all these cases, only 1 paced and 10 nonpaced patients were discharged.

Two-thirds (404) had known down time to ACLS data: 63 of 119 (53%) of paced and 129 of 285 (45%) of nonpaced had down time to ACLS under 8 minutes. This subset of patients with known down time to ACLS under 8 minutes was further compared for survival (Fig. 6). Of 63 paced patients, 61 (97%) died, 2 (3%) were admitted, and none survived to discharge. In the nonpaced control group, 125 of 129 patients (97%) died, 4 (3%) were admitted, and 3 (2%) were discharged alive (p = NS). For arrests with known down time over 8 minutes, 1 of 56 paced and 2 of 156 control patients were admitted. None of either group survived to discharge (p = NS).

Time from receipt of call to arrival at hospital was compared (Table 3). Paced patients averaged 38.45 minutes and controls 31.95 minutes (p< = 0.0005). Resuscitated patients averaged 41.6 minutes in the paced group and 31.1 minutes in the control group. Paced patients

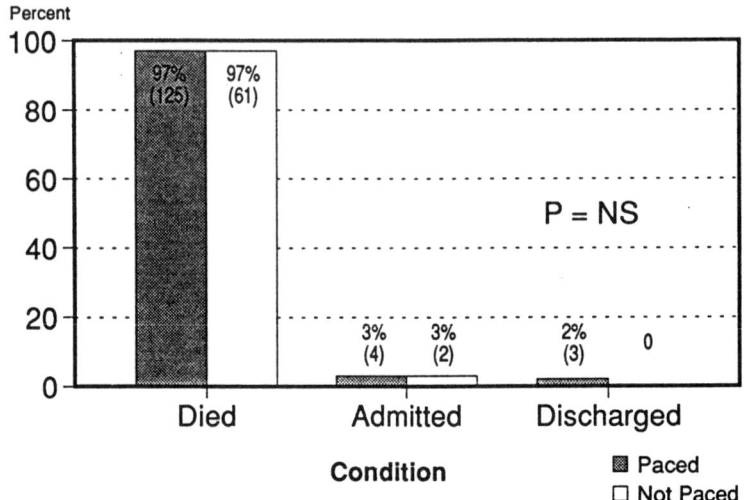

Figure 6: *Survival for arrests with known time to ACLS under 8 mn.*

Table 3. Time in Field Until Arrival At Hospital and Outcome for Paced and Control Patients

	Paced	Not Paced	Significance
All Patients	38.5 min	32.0 min	P<.0005
Admitted	41.6 min	31.1 min	NS
Pronounced	38.2 min	32.1 min	NS
Discharged	46.8 min	29.7 min	NS

who were pronounced in the emergency department (ED) averaged 38.2 minutes and controls 32.1 minutes (p=NS). Of patients discharged from the hospital, paced averaged 46.8 minutes in the field while controls were 29.7 minutes. While there was a difference in the field times, this did not correlate significantly with outcomes (p=NS).

Discussion

Assuming a survival rate of 6% with current therapy and looking for an 80% chance ($\beta = 0.80$ for type II error) of detecting a 10% difference in survival using a one-tailed test with significance level of

5% ($p < = 0.05$) accepted, a sample size of 121 patients in each study arm was needed to detect a benefit. The overall sample size of 145 paced and 376 nonpaced patients was adequate. In this situation, it appears unnecessary to rule out statistically a detrimental effect with a two-tailed test. Data is missing for certain parameters evaluated and thus lowered the total number of cases that can be compared for that particular category of data. Cases comprising the individual rhythm subgroups were too few in number when all asystolic cases were eliminated to be of actual clinical or statistical significance.

This controlled prospective prehospital trial of NTCP did not identify a significant improvement with respect to presentation to the emergency department with a pulse or blood pressure, admission to the hospital, or survival to hospital discharge with the use of prehospital pacing. No difference was shown for individual rhythms in pacer response.

Duration of arrest prior to the start of pacing was not able to be determined on enough cases to merit evaluation. However, because rapid response time and ACLS treatment early in arrest are known to improve survival chances, a subset of patients with known time to ACLS under 8 minutes from down time was evaluated. This group also did not show any clinically or statistically significant survival difference.

Although interesting, it was not statistically significant that more nonpaced patients (7%) in this study actually survived to discharge than paced ones (3%). Paced patients averaged 6.5 minutes longer in the field from receipt of ambulance call to arrival at the emergency department than nonpaced patients. There was, however, no correlation with outcome. Delays in the field observed in the pacing cases can be attributed principally to the multiplicity of other tasks to be done in the field by only two or three paramedics at the scene. The task of pacing must be accomplished along with intubation, CPR, IV access, and telemetry contact.

Questions remain regarding patient population subsets that might benefit from NTCP. In the prehospital setting, it is inappropriate and impractical for paramedics to attempt to diagnose the clinical cause of a specific dysrhythmia to then determine possible pacing usefulness in select cases. Furthermore, limiting its scope of application or use to the few patients that may eventually be identified that would benefit also includes the risk that this limited, rare application of NTCP by paramedics will lead to loss of pacing skills.

The use of a combined pacer-defibrillator-monitor would eliminate the problem of extra equipment to carry and hook up, as well as contribute to a possible reduction in pacing delay. The development of a practical, affordable combined pacer-defibrillator and monitor pad could further eliminate delays due to the current use of multiple pads for each function. It remains to be shown, however, that NTCP is useful in the prehospital setting and that it warrants the added equipment expense, no matter how convenient the combined equipment design.

Conclusion

Many articles tout the merits of prehospital NTCP and paramedic systems are adopting it, yet only three studies used comparison groups. None recorded numerically meaningful benefits. We report a two-year prospective controlled trial of external pacing in an advanced life support paramedic system with mean response time of 3.9 ± 3.3 minutes to evaluate its use. The study population consisted of 604 adults (73 ± 14 years old) with nontraumatic hemodynamically significant bradycardia, pulseless idioventricular rhythm or asystole not responsive to initial Advanced Cardiac Life Support care. Based on a systematic allocation of the pacers, nonpaced patients served as controls. Eleven pacers rotated monthly on eight ambulances. Of 228 patients with pacer availability, 145 were paced. In 59%, capture was noted, 14% had pulses, 7% were admitted, and 3% were discharged. Of the 459 nonpaced patients, 12% regained pulses with standard ACLS care, 11% were admitted and 7% were discharged. There was no statistically significant difference or outcome variables by rhythm, or time to ACLS care. All groups were comparable for age, sex, witnessed events, response time, and time to ACLS.

Given the results of other controlled studies and the absence of any outcome benefit of NTCP in bradyasystole in this trial, we believe that to advocate such is premature and possibly ill-advised.

Acknowledgments: This research was supported in part by a Health Research grant of $30,200.00 from Allstate Insurance Co., Northbrook, Illinois. Additional recognition to: Cardiac Resuscitator Corporation, Portland, Oregon for donation of PACE AID®, Model 53 pacemakers and carrying cases used during the study; Dr. Maria Norusis, Department of Preventive Medicine, Rush-Presbyterian-St. Luke's Hospitals, Chicago, Illinois for statistical analysis; Dr. Tom Reminga, Chairman, Department of Emergency Medicine, Columbia Hospital, Milwaukee, Wisconsin for computer database programming; MaryAnn Marcotte, RN, Director of Paramedic Training, St. Francis Emergency Medical Services System for paramedic training and promotion of the study; and Ms. Corinne Chan for data entry.

References

1. Tweed WA, Bristow G, Donen N: Resuscitation from cardiac arrest: Assessment of a system providing only basic life support outside of hospital. Can Med J 122:297, 1980.
2. Myerberg RJ, Kessler KM, Zaman L, et al.: Survivors of prehospital cardiac arrest. JAMA 247:1485, 1982.
3. Eisenberg M, Hallstrom A, Bergner L.: The ACLS Score: Predicting survival from out-of-hospital arrest. JAMA 246:50, 1981.
4. Sowden GR, Robins DW, Basket PJF.: Factors associated with survival and eventual cerebral status following cardiac arrest. Anaesthesia 39:39, 1984.
5. Scott RPF: Cardiopulmonary resuscitation in a teaching hospital. A survey of cardiac arrests occuring outside intensive care units and emergency room. Anaesthesia 36:526, 1981.
6. Wernberg W, Thomassen A: Prognosis after cardiac arrest occurring outside intensive care and coronary units. Acta Anaesthesiol Scand 23:69, 1979.
7. Baldwin M, Iverson RL: Cardio-pulmonary resuscitation: does it work? Indiana Med 77:246, 1984.
8. Syverud SA, Dalsey WC, Hedges JR: Transcutaneous and transvenous cardiac pacing for early bradyasystolic cardiac arrest. Ann Emerg Med 15:121, 1986.
9. McNeil EL: Successful resuscitation using external cardiac pacing. Ann Emerg Med 14:1230, 1985.
10. Zoll PM, Zoll RH, Falk RH, et al.: External noninvasive temporary cardiac pacing: Clinical trials. Circulation 71:937, 1985.
11. White JM, Nowak RM, Martin GB, et al.: Immediate emergency department external cardiac pacing for prehospital bradyasystolic pacing arrest. Ann Emerg Med 14:298, 1985.
12. Dalsey WC, Syverud SA, Hedges JR: Emergency department use of transcutaneous pacing for cardiac arrests. Crit Care Med 13:399, 1985.
13. O'Connor R, Reese C, Lombardi A, et al.: Use of transcutaneous cardiac pacing in the emergency department for treatment of prehospital bradyasystolic cardiopulmonary arrest (abstr). Ann Emerg Med 14:501, 1985.
14. Zoll PM, Zoll RH: Noninvasive temporary cardiac stimulation. Crit Care Med 13:925, 1985.
15. Altamura G, Toscano S, Lo Bianco F, et al.: Emergency cardiac pacing for severe bradycardia. PACE 16 (part II):2038, 1990.
16. Heber M: Out-of-hospital resuscitation using the "heart aid," an automated external defibrillator-pacemaker. Int J Cardiol 3:456, 1983.

17. Diack AW, Welborn WS, Rullman RG, et al.: An automatic cardiac resuscitator for emergency treatment of cardiac arrest. Med Instrum 13:78, 1979.
18. Leatham A, Cook P, Davies JG: External electric stimulator for treatment of ventricular standstill. Lancet, 271:1185, 1956.
19. Zoll PM, Linenthal AJ, Norman LR, et al.: Use of external electric pacemaker in cardiac arrest. JAMA, 159:1428, 1955.
20. Zoll PM, Linenthal AJ, Norman LR, et al.: External electric stimulation of the heart in cardiac arrest. Arch Int Med 96:639, 1955.
21. Zoll PM: Resuscitation of the heart in ventricular standstill by external electrical stimulation. N Engl J Med 247:768, 1952.
22. Callaghan JC, Bigelow WG: An electric artificial pacemaker for standstill of the heart. Ann Surg, 134:8, 1951.
23. Madsen JK, Meibom J, Videbak R, et al.: Transcutaneous pacing: Experience with the Zoll noninvasive temporary pacemaker. Am Heart J 116 (Part I):7, 1988.
24. Vukov LF, Johnson DQ: External transcutaneous pacemakers in interhospital transport of cardiac patients. Ann Emerg Med 18:738, 1989.
25. National Conference on Pulmonary Resuscitation and Emergency Cardiac Care: Standards and Guidelines for Cardiopulmonary Resuscitation and Emergency Cardiac Care. JAMA 255:2948, 1986.
26. Syverud SA, Dalsey WC, Hedges JR, et al.: Transcutaneous cardiac pacing: determination of myocardial injury in a canine model. Ann Emerg Med 12:745, 1983.
27. Hedges JR, Syverud SA, Dalsey WC, et al.: Prehospital trial of emergency transcutaneous cardiac pacing. Circulation 76:1337, 1987.
28. Barthell E, Troiano P, Olso, D, et al.: Prehospital external cardiac pacing: a prospective, controlled clinical trial. Ann Emerg Med 17:1221, 1988.
29. Jaggarao NSV, Heber M, Grainger R, et al.: Use of automated external defibrillator-pacemaker by ambulance staff. Lancet 2:73, 1982.
30. Falk RH, Jacobs L, Sinclair A, et al.: External noninvasive cardiac pacing in an out-of-hospital cardiac arrest. Crit Care Med 11:779, 1983.
31. Paris PM, Stewart RD, Kaplan R, et al.: Transcutaneous pacing for bradyasystolic cardiac arrests in prehospital care. Ann Emerg Med 14:320, 1985.
32. Eitel DR, Guzzardi LR, Stein SE, et al.: Noninvasive transcutaneous cardiac pacing in prehospital cardiac arrest. Ann Emerg Med 16:531, 1987.
33. O'Toole KS, Paris PM, Heller MB, et al.: Emergency transcutaneous pacing in the management of patients with bradyasystolic rhythms. J Emerg Med 5:267, 1987.
34. Hedges JR, Feero S, Easter R, et al.: Prehospital transcutaneous cardiac pacing—Phase II (abstr). Ann Emerg Med 13:469, 1989.
35. Kennedy RS: Clinical investigations with medical devices. JAMA 245:2052, 1981.

V

Application in Children

Chapter 8

Noninvasive Transcutaneous Cardiac Pacing in Children

Marie J. Beland, MDCM, FRCPC

Prior to the development and refinement of transcutaneous pacing, transvenous and transthoracic pacing were the only methods available for emergency temporary ventricular pacing. The establishment of ventricular capture by these methods is time-consuming, requires specially trained personnel, and is fraught with potential complications,[1,2] particularly in smaller children.[3] Noninvasive transcutaneous cardiac pacing (NTCP), on the other hand, can be instituted swiftly and with little risk. This section will review the clinical aspects of NTCP in children including technique, risk, and indications.

Technique

Preparing the Child

Prior to initiating transcutaneous pacing in children, sedation, intubation, and artificial ventilation should be considered.

Transcutaneous pacing is seldom possible in the unsedated child because of difficulties with patient cooperation due to the mild to moderate discomfort associated with this pacing modality. In addition to sedation, smaller children are likely to require artificial ventilation during NTCP. Compared to adults, the pacing pads cover a relatively

From *Noninvasive Transcutaneous Cardiac Pacing* edited by Pierre Birkui, M.D., Jacques Trigano, M.D., and Paul Zoll, M.D., © 1993, Futura Publishing Company, Inc., Mount Kisco, NY.

large area of a child's thorax. This results in more extensive skeletal muscle stimulation during pacing which can hamper spontaneous ventilation, especially in infants. Thus, intubation is often required during NTCP in younger patients.

If the patient is intubated, neuromuscular blockade should also be considered during NTCP to facilitate assisted ventilation by eliminating skeletal muscle contractions. Neuromuscular blockade can have the added benefit of making the electrocardiographic tracing less difficult to interpret by decreasing movement artefact during pacing.

Electrode Placement

The positioning of the transcutaneous electrode pads in the pediatric population does not differ from that in adults. The pads should be placed over the area of the cardiac mass both anteriorly and posteriorly (Fig. 1). They should be positioned over the right hemitho-

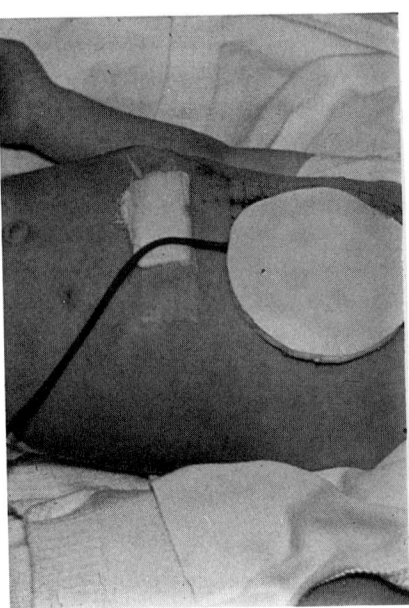 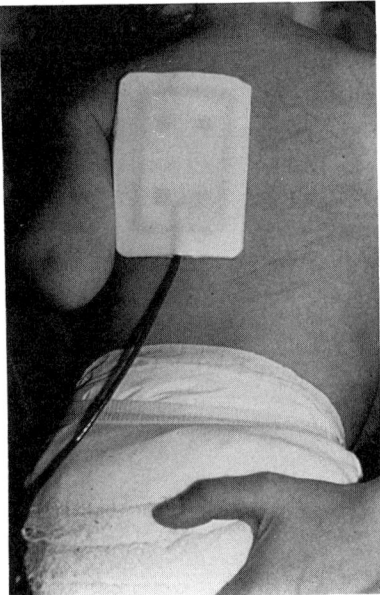

Figure 1. *Pediatric electrode placement on an 8 kg child after cardiac surgery. Left: anterior pad is placed to the left of the sternum. Right: posterior pad is positioned to the left of the vertebral column.*

rax in patients with dextrocardia, or more toward the midline in children with mesocardia.

Electrode Pad Size

In a study involving 22 anesthetized pediatric patients and three electrode sizes, it was noted that as the electrode size increases, the pacing threshold increases, but the current density delivered at threshold decreases.[4] Because current density is probably the most important determinant of patient comfort and risk of thermal injury, the largest size electrodes that will fit over the cardiac mass without overlapping the neck and abdomen should be used.

Standard anterior circular electrodes of 10 cm in diameter are unlikely to be suitable for children weighing less than 15 kg because they tend to extend beyond the thorax and cover the neck and abdomen. Electrodes that are too large relative to the patient's size will cause more extensive skeletal muscle stimulation. They will also fail to adhere properly giving rise to difficulties in obtaining good patient-electrode contact and reliable capture. For these reasons, smaller pediatric electrode pads have been developed and are recommended for children under 15 kg, while standard "adult" pads can be used in children weighing more than 15 kg.

Pacing Threshold

In the study mentioned above involving patients from 0.9 to 18 years of age, mean output at threshold is reported as 63 ± 14 mA (range: 42 to 98 mA) using standard pads (virtually identical to postanesthetic thresholds described in adults,[5] and 51 ± 11 mA (range: 29 to 82 mA) with the smaller pediatric pads.[4] Interestingly, age, body surface area, weight, and chest circumference (Fig. 2) did not alter current requirements in this group of children. No child required more than 100 mA to obtain successful capture, regardless of the pad size used.

As in adults, pacing threshold should be established prior to, or at the onset of, sustained transcutaneous pacing. Capture is recognized on the NTCP monitor by the demonstration of a pacing artefact followed by QRS and T waves of a different morphology than that of the spontaneous QRS and T waves of the patient (Fig. 3). Because

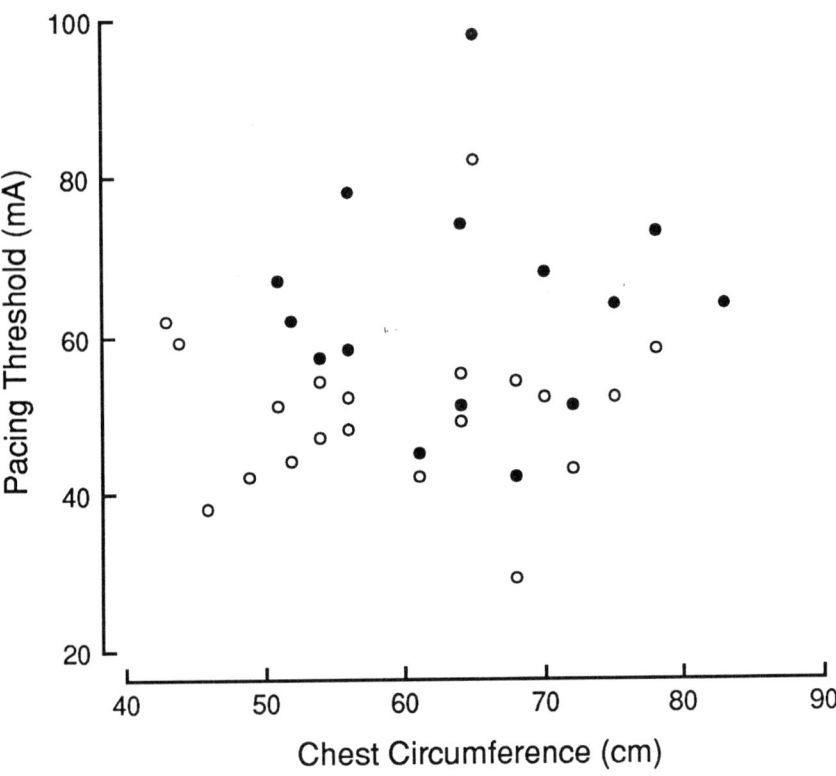

Figure 2. *In a study of NTCP in pediatric patients, no correlation could be found between chest circumference (range: 43 to 83 cm), and pacing thresholds. Solid circles = pacing thresholds obtained with standard "adult" electrode size. Open circles = pacing thresholds using the smaller pediatric electrodes.*

Noninvasive Transcutaneous Cardiac Pacing in Children

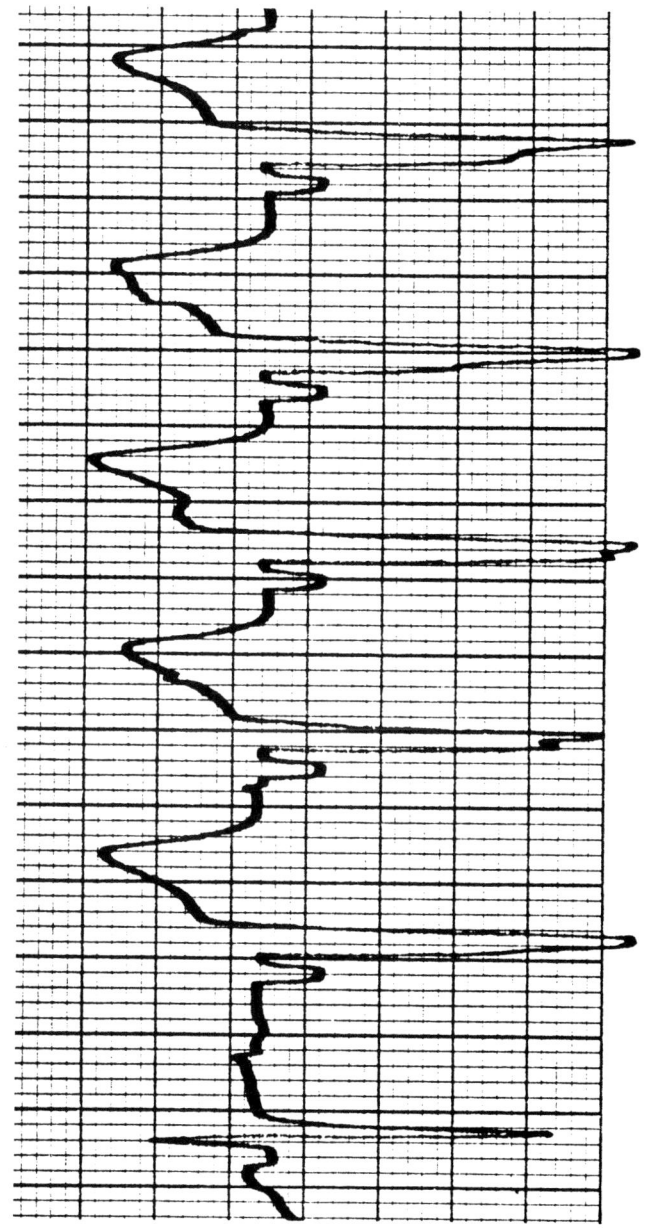

Figure 3. Rhythm strip during NTCP: a spontaneous QRS is followed by five paced ventricular beats preceded by a box-like pacing artefact.

regular ECG monitor tracings are greatly distorted by the pacemaker artefact, tracings are best obtained via monitors that contain special amplifiers which will specifically dampen the pacing signal. As long as there is electrical-mechanical association, capture can also be ascertained indirectly by an increase in the heart rate as detected by a peripheral arterial tracing or by Doppler monitoring of a peripheral pulse.

Risks

Transcutaneous pacing has generally been considered a safe method of emergency ventricular pacing. Three reports (including one involving a three-year-old child) have described arrhythmias associated with transcutaneous pacing.[6-8] Continuous ECG monitoring is mandatory and a defibrillator should be on standby during NTCP.

It is not unusual for transcutaneous pacing to cause transient reddening of the skin under the electrode pads. This usually resolves within minutes of stopping NTCP. Although there have been no published reports of thermal injuries secondary to transcutaneous pacing, skin burns have been known to occur in neonates with congenital complete heart block being paced for greater than 30 mn. This may be due to a particular sensitivity of newborn skin combined with the fact that a larger current density must be delivered to achieve capture when using the smaller pediatric pads. In newborns and infants, it is therefore recommended that the area under the pads should be inspected regularly during pacing to ensure that pronounced erythema suggestive of a burn has not appeared.

Indications

The following list outlines potential indications for transcutaneous pacemaker use in children, either on standby or for emergency use:

1. In patients who are dependent on temporary epicardial pacing after surgery for congenital heart disease, in case of failure of the temporary pacemaker or problems with the epicardial wires;

2. During permanent pacemaker reprogramming in pacemaker-dependent patients during routine clinic visits;
3. During general anesthesia in patients with complete heart block;
4. In patients suffering from intoxication with drugs which may result in severe bradycardia or A-V block;
5. To treat long pauses after cardioversion in patients with sick sinus syndrome, particularly patients who have undergone the atrial switch repair (Mustard or Senning operations) for transposition of the great arteries;
6. In patients with symptomatic complete heart block while awaiting permanent pacemaker placement.

Most severe bradycardias or cardiac arrests in children are the result of acute hypoxia and problems with ventilation. They respond to prompt airway support and maintenance with or without drug therapy. Thus unlike adults, transcutaneous pacing is rarely required in an arrest situation in pediatrics.

Future Indications for Transcutaneous Pacing

Presently, the design of commercially-available devices does not allow for programmed stimulation with synchronized extrastimuli or burst pacing at rates greater than 180 ppm. However, several investigators have successfully terminated supraventricular and ventricular tachycardias using programmed transcutaneous stimulation or overdrive pacing by modifying the pacemaker devices.[9,10] This application is less likely to gain favor in pediatrics because of the responsiveness of reentry supraventricular tachycardias to medical treatment or transesophageal pacing, and because of the need for premedication and assisted ventilation during NTCP in younger children.

Conclusion

Transcutaneous cardiac pacing in children is a rapid, effective, and relatively safe technique for ventricular pacing. Little difference exists between transcutaneous pacing in the child and the adult. However, premedications, electrode pad size, and possible risks specific to the pediatric age group must be considered prior to NTCP in children.

References

1. Tintinalli JE, White BC: Transthoracic pacing during CPR. Ann Emerg Med 10:113, 1981.
2. Hazard PB, Benton C, Milnor JP: Transvenous cardiac pacing in cardiopulmonary resuscitation. Crit Care Med 9:666, 1981.
3. So LY, Sung RYT, Ho JKS, et al.: Management of a hydropic infant with congenital heart block. J Paediatr Child Health 26:158, 1990.
4. Béland MJ, Hesslein PS, Finlay CD, et al.: Noninvasive transcutaneous cardiac pacing in children. PACE 10:1262, 1987.
5. Kelly JS, Royster RL, Angert KC, et al.: Efficacy of noninvasive transcutaneous cardiac pacing in patients undergoing cardiac surgery. Anesthesiology 70:747, 1989.
6. Béland MJ, Hesslain PS, Rowe RD: Ventricular tachycardia related to transcutaneous pacing for cardiac arrests. Ann Emerg Med 17:279, 1988.
7. Dalsey WC, Syverud SA, Hedges JR: Emergency department use of transcutaneous pacing for cardiac arrests. Crit Care Med 13:399, 1985.
8. Feldman MD, Zoll PM, Aroesty JM, et al.: Hemodynamic responses to noninvasive external cardiac pacing. Am J Med 84:395, 1988.
9. Estes NAM, Deering TF, Manolis AS, et al.: External cardiac programmed stimulation for noninvasive termination of sustained supraventricular tachycardia. Am J Cardiol 63:177, 1989.
10. Luck JC, Grubb BP, Artman SE, et al.: Termination of sustained ventricular tachycardia by external noninvasive pacing. Am J Cardiol 61:574, 1988.

VI

Progress in Clinical Electrophysiology

Chapter 9

Noninvasive Cardiac Stimulation, Fibrillation, and Defibrillation

Paul M. Zoll, MD, Ross H. Zoll, MD, PhD

With increasing knowledge of the physics and technology of electricity in the nineteenth century, understanding of its cardiac effects also developed. In 1887, J.A. MacWilliam[1] described fibrillary contractions of the heart and identified ventricular fibrillation as a major mechanism of cardiac arrest. He also described the much lower thresholds for stimulating the exposed heart in animals.[2] In 1890, J.L. Prevost and F. Batelli produced ventricular fibrillation in the exposed chest preparation with electric shocks of both direct and alternating current.[3] They then demonstrated that shocks slightly above fibrillating threshold would defibrillate the heart.

From 1925 to 1950, Carl Wiggers greatly advanced our knowledge of cardiac responses to electric currents in open-chest experiments in animals:[4] "shocks" would stimulate single or multiple beats or produce fibrillation and larger "countershocks" would terminate fibrillation. He taught that emergency thoracotomy would be necessary through which to apply sufficient current to the exposed heart to terminate ventricular fibrillation, and that currents large enough to do so across the closed chest wall would be fatal. Indeed in 1947, the use of emergency thoracotomy, cardiac massage, and direct countershock was introduced by Claude Beck,[5] who even suggested later that such resuscitations should be attempted not only by physicians in hospitals but by laymen anywhere.

From *Noninvasive Transcutaneous Cardiac Pacing* edited by Pierre Birkui, M.D., Jacques Trigano, M.D., and Paul Zoll, M.D., © 1993, Futura Publishing Company, Inc., Mount Kisco, NY.

Early in 1932 Albert Hyman,[6] an outstanding New York City cardiologist, developed a cardiac pacemaker from which he passed electric stimuli to the atrium, initially in rabbits, via a long transthoracic needle. Although several patients were ultimately resuscitated, the cases were not published because of concern over local ethical and religious objections.

In 1950, Bigelow and Callaghan attempted to stimulate the heart with an endocardial wire electrode passed to the sino-atrial node after intervals of cardiac arrest due to hypothermia that might be prolonged enough to provide sufficient time for cardiac surgery.[7] Their attempts failed, apparently because their electrode was placed short of the S-A node.

In 1950, my interest in cardiac resuscitation was rekindled following the death of a patient under my care despite all desperate measures from recurring Stokes-Adams attacks over a three-week interval. My initial thought was to stimulate the heart by way of a negative esophageal electrode behind the heart and a small positive one on the surface over the apex. At the suggestion of Dr. Callaghan, I used a Grass physiological thyratron pulse generator that was effective in stimulating ventricular response in laboratory animals. In fact, it was so effective that I soon used two electrodes externally, one on each side of the chest wall, to stimulate the heart as a clinically quicker and a more useful procedure than esophageal pacing. We then waited for appropriate patients with severe Stokes-Adams attacks. Two patients appeared a month apart in 1952, the first being stimulated effectively for 20 minutes until he died of cardiac tamponade from previously inserted needles, and the second who was resuscitated after 52 hours of almost continuous stimulation.[8] Shortly thereafter, I worked with the small Electrodyne Company to develop a pulse generator smaller than the Grass unit. These units were widely used for years and, indeed, were successful in producing ventricular responses noninvasively to treat Stokes-Adams disease and other bradycardias and asystoles. They did, however, usually cause considerable pain from an electrical sting and burning sensation of the skin and from severe muscular contractions. It was also difficult to read electrocardiograms because of large electrical artefacts and skeletal muscular contractions concurrent with the stimuli. The technique of noninvasive cardiac pacing gained wide acceptance for temporary purposes in resuscitating patients from arrest with effective beats until intrinsic ventricular rhythm returned. Noninvasive pacemakers were widely used not only to provide effective heart beats and to restore intrinsic rhythm, but also to suppress ectopy and tachycardia by acceleration of the heart rate.

Efforts were then made to develop obviously needed long-term, permanently implanted cardiac pacemakers to protect patients indefinitely. Many serious difficulties with the new, complicated technology delayed their appearance for almost ten years.

An additional problem associated with bradycardias and heart block was the need for constant observation of rhythm to avoid delay in identifying mortal arrhythmias, so as to resuscitate patients in the very short time available. Cardiac monitors were developed that would watch electrocardiographic patterns continuously on an oscilloscopic screen, ring a loud alarm, and permit prompt identification of rhythm to facilitate prompt effective treatment.[9] Resuscitation was particularly successful in hospitalized patients already being monitored. Cardiac monitors became widely used, particularly in conjunction with noninvasive pacemakers and defibrillators.

Noninvasive defibrillators were then developed that would terminate ventricular fibrillation and other tachycardias as well. Initially, they contained large 60-cycle alternating-current transformers that would provide 0.15 second shocks up to 720 volts in amplitude. Later, they were combined with external noninvasive pacemakers and monitors, and the first successful noninvasive alternating-current defibrillation was accomplished in 1956.[10] In the laboratory, techniques were developed to produce every kind of tachycardia in canine and pig models, and then to demonstrate their successful termination with noninvasive defibrillation ("shock and countershock"). One of our first patients with recurrent ventricular tachycardia was successfully restored to sinus rhythm in 1962.[11]

In 1963, Hughes Day organized the first coronary care unit in which noninvasive pacemakers, monitors, and defibrillators were applied by physicians and nurses skilled in their use to treat patients with acute myocardial infarction and serious arrhythmias. His demonstration of a striking, improved survival of such patients led to the widespread establishment of these specialized units with their specialized equipment.

Shortly thereafter, other direct-current defibrillators became available in many variations to terminate recurrent arrhythmias. Several types of capacitor discharges were used (underdamped, overdamped, truncated trapezoidal). Synchronized countershock termination of arrhythmias to avoid stimulation in the "vulnerable" period of the cardiac cycle was renamed cardioversion instead of countershock.

In 1958, the first cardiac long-term pacemaker was implanted by Ake Senning.[12] Subsequently, endocardial electrodes, introduced pervenously by Furman[13] to avoid the more formidable thoracotomies previously required, were attached to external pacemakers. They were later connected to small implanted pulse generators to provide totally implanted systems and the promise of long-term durability. Endocardial placement of electrodes was also often used for temporary purposes even though they were not suitable for emergencies, primarily because of the excessive time involved. They were used to avoid the frequent severe discomfort that noninvasive external pacing usually entailed. Over the years, noninvasive pacing was largely displaced for that reason by temporary endocardial electrodes despite their tendency toward displacement, hemorrhage, thrombosis, infection, and even ventricular fibrillation.[14]

In 1976, a mechanical thumping machine was developed in an attempt to provide noninvasive pacing without significant discomfort.[15] This instrument was useful initially, particularly for special brief applications, but rather quickly was found, with prolonged use, to produce too much tissue discomfort from mechanical trauma.

In 1980, modifications were made in noninvasive temporary pacing in many different aspects so as to reduce the pain of stimulation and to provide clearer recordings of the cardiac events.[16] Changes were made in the pulse duration, shape, and amplitude of the stimuli, and composition of the electrodes that reduced the amplitude of the current threshold for stimulation in terms of milliamperes so as largely to eliminate the sting and burning pain of the skin, and also to reduce the remaining muscular contractions significantly.[17] Extensive laboratory tests were required to assure that these changes, particularly the prolongation of the pulse duration, did not narrow the "safety factor," or the ratio of threshold for producing serious arrhythmias over the threshold for stimulating single beats. As predicted by the tests, no such untoward arrhythmias have occurred.

In addition, the monitoring systems of the pacemakers were modified to present an unmistakable symbol to identify a stimulus artefact and its exact timing, and to isolate the recording on screen and paper from the relatively large and prolonged current wave introduced into the body by each stimulus. The disturbing current was also minimized by means of a "blanking interval" in the monitor circuitry that coincides with each stimulus. Similarly, noninvasive defibrillators with monitors, and then combined noninvasive pacemaker-defibrillator-monitor units, were developed in the same format as the single-purpose instruments. They present a noninvasive pacemaker, defibrillator, and monitor in one familiar unit with multifunctional electrodes that provide prompt stimulation, defibrillation, or countershock termination of arrhythmias as needed. These instruments are particularly useful in the not infrequent instances when defibrillation is followed by ventricular standstill. The monitor recorder presents on paper and screen detailed recordings of all electric manipulations and easy recognition of electrocardiographic responses to them. Many new uses are being developed in termination of arrhythmias with these versatile instruments that are safe, noninvasive, and quick and easy to use. The most recent model, a small, combined unit weighing only fifteen pounds, is shown below (Fig. 1).

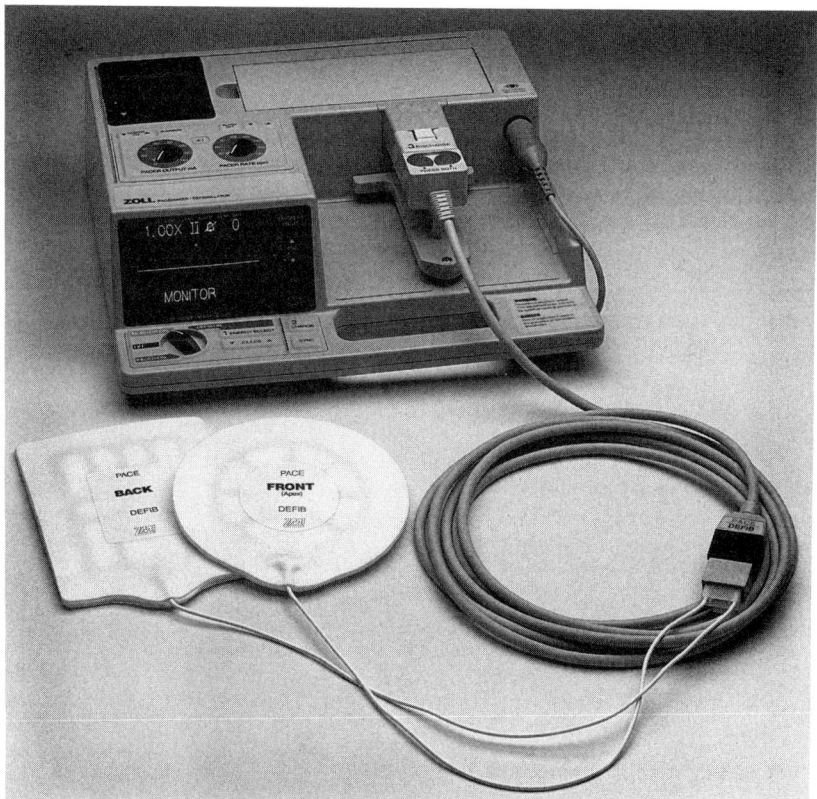

Figure 1. *Recent model of noninvasive pacing and "hands off" defibrillation with a single set of prejelled disposable electrodes.*

References

1. MacWilliam JA: Fibrillar contraction of the heart. J Physiol 8:296, 1887.
2. MacWilliam JA: Electrical stimulation of the mammalian heart. Tr Internat M Congr 3:253, 1887.
3. Prevost JL, Batelli F: La mort par les déchargesy électriques. J Physiol Pathol Gén 1:1085, 1899.
4. Wiggers CJ, Wegria R: Ventricular fibrillation due to single, localized induction and condenser shocks applied during the vulnerable phase of ventricular systole. Amer J Physiol 128:500, 1940.
5. Beck CS, Pritchard WH, Feil HS: Ventricular fibrillation of long duration abolished by electric shock. JAMA 135:985, 1947.
6. Hyman AS: Resuscitation of the stopped heart by intracardial therapy. II. Experimental use of an artificial pacemaker. Arch Intern Med 50:283, 1932.
7. Bigelow WG, Callaghan JC, Hopps JA: General hypothermia for experimental intracardiac surgery. The use of electrophrenic respirations, an artificial pacemaker for cardiac standstill, and radio-frequency rewarming in general hypothermia. Ann Surg 132:531, 1950.
8. Zoll PM: Resuscitation of the heart in ventricular standstill by external electrical stimulation. N Engl J Med 247:768, 1952.
9. Zoll PM, Linenthal AJ, Norman LR, et al.: Treatment of unexpected cardiac arrest by external electric stimulation of the heart. N Engl J Med 254:541, 1956.
10. Zoll PM, Linenthal AJ, Gibson W, et al.: Termination of ventricular fibrillation in man by externally applied electric countershock. N Engl J Med 254:727, 1956.
11. Zoll PM, Linenthal AJ: Termination of refractory tachycardia by external countershock. Circulation 225:596, 1962.
12. Senning A: Discussion. J Thor Surg 38:639, 1959.
13. Furman S, Robinson G: The use of an intracardiac pacemaker in the correction of total heart block. Surg Forum 9:245, 1958.
14. Austin JL, Preis LK, Crampton RS, et al.: Analysis of pacemaker malfunction and complications of temporary pacing in the coronary care unit. Am J Cardiol 49:301, 1982.
15. Zoll PM, Belgard AH, Weintraub MD, et al.: External mechanical cardiac stimulation. N Engl J Med 294:1274, 1976.
16. Zoll RH, Zoll PM, Belgard AH: External noninvasive electric stimulation of the heart. Crit Care Med 9:393, 1981.
17. Zoll PM, Zoll RH, Falk RH, et al.: External noninvasive temporary cardiac pacing: Clinical trials. Circulation 71:937, 1985.

Chapter 10

Noninvasive Transcutaneous Cardiac Pacing for Termination of Ventricular and Supraventricular Tachycardias

Giuliano Altamura, MD, Leopoldo Bianconi, MD, Salvatore Toscano, MD, Francesco Lo Bianco, MD, Massimo Santini, MD

Underdrive or overdrive pacing and programmed electrical stimulation are all well established techniques apt to interrupt different kinds of reentrant ventricular and supraventricular tachyarrhythmias.[1-5]

The reintroduction of the noninvasive transcutaneous cardiac pacing (NTCP) in the emergency treatment of the bradyarrhythmias at the beginning of the 1980s, has raised the possibility of testing this technique for the termination of ventricular (VT) and supraventricular tachycardias (SVT). Since the use of NTCP in this clinical setting is attractive due to its simple, rapid, and noninvasive utilization, we report our up-to-date experience in this field, together with a review of the literature today available on this topic.

Material and Methods

NTCP was employed in 36 patients with spontaneous sustained tachyarrhythmias: 20 monomorphic ventricular tachycardias, 10

From *Noninvasive Transcutaneous Cardiac Pacing* edited by Pierre Birkui, M.D., Jacques Trigano, M.D., and Paul Zoll, M.D., © 1993, Futura Publishing Company, Inc., Mount Kisco, NY.

atrioventricular reentrant tachycardias (6 concealed atrioventricular bypass tract and 4 Wolff-Parkinson-White syndrome), 3 intranodal reentrant tachycardias, and 3 atrial flutter. The hemodynamic conditions of the patients were stable enough to allow the noninvasive pacing procedure to be performed.

The diagnosis of ventricular tachycardia was initially based on the usual surface ECG criteria.[6] In 13 cases, it was possible thereafter to confirm the diagnosis by electrophysiological study. In the patients with supraventricular tachycardias, the site of the reentrant pathway (atrioventricular or intranodal) was based on a complete electrophysiological study in five patients and on electrocardiographic criteria[7] in the remaining cases.

The cardiopathies associated with ventricular tachycardias were: acute myocardial infarction in five cases, chronic ischemic heart disease in ten, dilated cardiomyopathy in three, and undetermined in two cases.

Two different transcutaneous stimulators (Cardiac Resuscitator Corporation, Oregon, USA) were used:

1. Pace Aid model 50, first device available to us, only used in the first four cases. This model has the following characteristics: asynchronous stimulation at the rate of 80 ppm, a pulse width of 20 msec, and three different pulse output energies (50, 100, 200 mA).
2. Pace Aid model 52. Unlike the former, it can also perform a demand stimulation at nine different programmable rates (50 to 160 ppm) and nine current output levels (from 10 to 150 mA).

A strip chart ECG recorder allows the registration of both the spontaneous and the paced cardiac electrical activity. The latter is made possible by introducing a blanking period after the emitted spike that permits the suppression of the recording distortion due to the high stimulation energy. The two cutaneous high impedance electrodes have a large surface area (50 cm^2), with a consequent low density current at the stimulation site.

The anterior electrode was applied at the ECG V_3 position and the posterior on the back at the cardiac level, between the left scapula and the spine.

For the interruption of the tachycardia, trains of asynchronous stimuli were delivered. The stimulation rates ranged from 80 to 160 ppm. Usually, we used the maximum pacing rate of the device but, due to its limited value, overdrive pacing was possible only for the slower tachycardias (six ventricular tachycardias, eight supraventricular tachycardias). Underdrive stimulation was used in all the remaining cases. In case of failure, each attempt was repeated at least three times, at each energy level delivered. In the last eight cases of supraventricular tachycardia, the maximum intensity current was employed directly at the first attempt.

Whenever possible, every patient was informed about the technique and the possible discomfort secondary to pacing, and asked to report the quality and the intensity of the sensation. The first attempts were carried out with medium intensity current, then the intensity was increased until the termination of the arrhythmia was obtained or the patient judged the stimulation intolerable.

Results (Table 1)

Ventricular tachycardia was interrupted by NTCP (Figs. 1, 2) in 8 of the 20 cases (40%). Underdrive pacing was used in 14 patients and it was successful in 4 (29%), while the tachycardia was interrupted in 4 of the 6 cases in which it was possible to perform an overdrive stimulation (67%). The mean ventricular rate was 191 ± 30 ppm in the cases treated by underdrive and 142 ± 11 ppm in those treated by

Table 1.

Patients	Overdrive N (%)	Underdrive N (%)	Total N (%)
VT	6	14	20
Interruption	4 (67)	4 (29)	8 (40)
AVRT	6	4	10
Interruption	6 (100)	2 (50)	8 (80)
AVNRT	2	2	4
Interruption	1 (50)	1 (50)	2 (50)
AF		3	3
Interruption		0	0

Interruption of ventricular and supraventricular tachycardias by NTP (overdrive or underdrive stimulation).
VT = ventricular tachycardia; AVRT = atrioventricular reentrant tachycardia; AVNRT = atrioventricular nodal reentrant tachycardia; AF = atrial flutter.

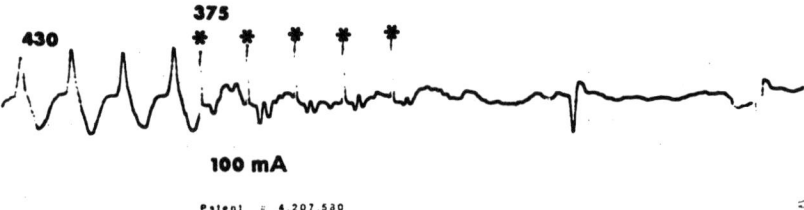

Figure 1. *Sustained ventricular tachycardia at 140 ppm (RR = 430 msec) terminated by 5 stimuli bursts at 160 ppm (SS = 375 msec), 100 mA.*

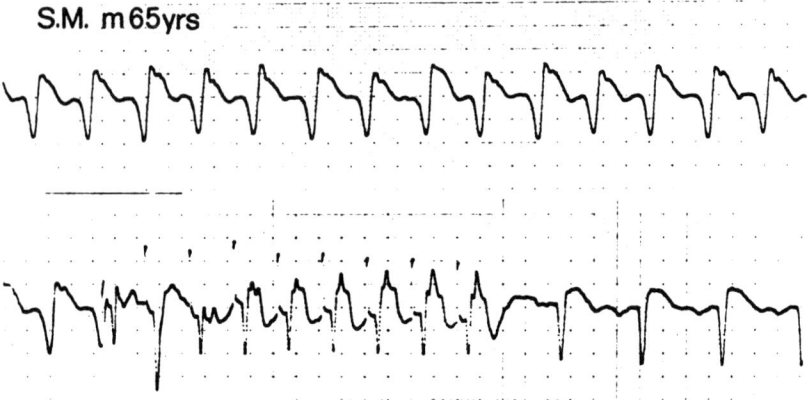

Figure 2. *(Continuous strip) Ventricular tachycardia (120 ppm) terminated by transcutaneous overdrive pacing (160 ppm).*

overdrive pacing (p<0.001). The mean pacing current effective in converters was 106 ± 29 mA.

Supraventricular reentrant tachycardias were terminated in 10 of the 14 cases (71%), usually by few stimuli at the first attempt (Figs. 3, 4). Atrioventricular reentrant tachycardias were interrupted more easily (8/10 = 80%) than the intranodal tachycardias (2/4 = 50%)(p = NS). Overdrive stimulation was effective in seven of eight cases (6/6 atrioventricular and 1/2 intranodal tachycardias), while underdrive stimulation terminated the arrhythmia in three of the six cases (2/4 atrioventricular and 1/2 intranodal tachycardias). The mean rate of SVT was 166 ± 21 ppm and the mean pacing current used in converters was 131 ± 32 mA.

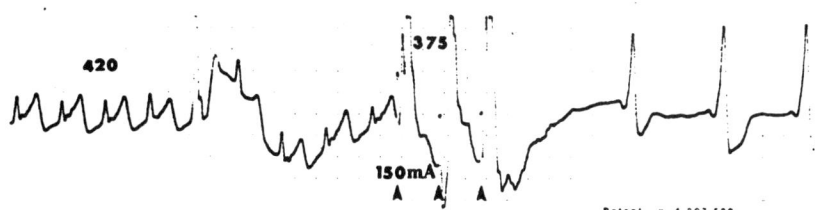

Figure 3. *Atrioventricular reentrant tachycardia at 145 ppm (RR = 420 msec) interrupted by 3 extrastimuli at 160 ppm (SS = 375 msec), 150mA. Resumption of sinus rhythm with ventricular preexcitation.*

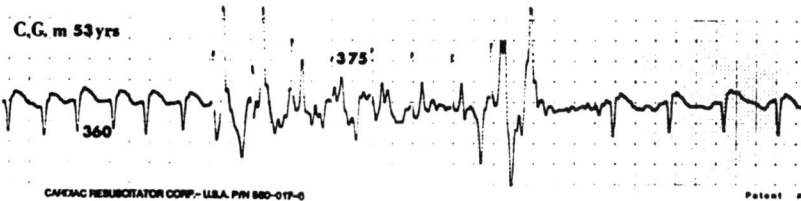

Figure 4. *Atrioventricular reentrant tachycardia at 165 ppm (RR = 360 msec), due to concealed bypass tract, interrupted by a burst of transcutaneous stimuli (SS = 375 msec).*

NTCP bursts at 160 ppm and 150 mA failed to interrupt atrial flutter in all the three cases in which it was tried.

All the patients reported an unpleasant sensation on the chest, usually described as a run of thumps, especially when high energies were used. Only 5 of the 18 patients in whom NTCP failed to interrupt the arrhythmia refused to try a stimulation at the maximum energy.

We observed two cases of arrhythmia worsening. In the first one, a ventricular tachycardia (150 ppm) was converted to a different morphology ventricular tachycardia (162 ppm), further unresponsive to subsequent NTCP attempts and finally converted by DC shock (Fig. 5). In the second patient affected by acute myocardial infarction and relapsing supraventricular intranodal tachycardia (180 ppm), inducing a low output syndrome and nonresponsive to different intravenous drugs (verapamil, digitalis, propafenone), short bursts of NTCP were repeatedly effective in restoring sinus rhythm. However, a last burst of three stimuli induced ventricular fibrillation requiring DC shock.

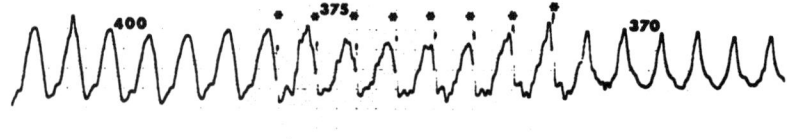

Figure 5. *Ventricular tachycardia at 150 ppm (RR = 400 msec). A burst of 8 stimuli at 160 ppm (SS = 375 msec), 80 mA, induces a different morphology ventricular tachycardia at 162 ppm (RR = 370 msec).*

Discussion

Low energy cardioversion, intravenous drugs or transvenous cardiac pacing are well established and effective methods for conversion of VT and SVT to normal rhythm. However, all of them have disadvantages. Cardioversion is very effective but can produce myocardial damage and requires anesthesia. Intravenous drugs can have serious drawbacks as negative inotropic action and proarrhythmic effects. Intracavitary pacing requires an invasive procedure and longer preparation times.

The possibility of terminating both ventricular and supraventricular reentrant tachycardias by a noninvasive, fast, and easily applicable technique as NTCP is undoubtedly attractive. The technique, well established in the emergency treatment of the bradyarrhythmias,[8] has been tested[8-16] in several tachyarrhythmias (Table 2). However, as can be deduced from the table, the experience is still scanty.

Pooling all the data available in the literature, NTCP resulted in successful termination of ventricular tachycardias in 75% (33/44) of the patients and supraventricular tachycardias in 86% (12/14). It was of no use in atrial flutter.

In the first report by Zoll,[8] NTCP was ineffective in case of "irregular ventricular tachycardia," in two cases of atrial tachycardia and in four cases of atrial flutter. Indeed, the stimulation protocol is not described and the type of atrial tachycardia is not specified. The failure to convert atrial flutter is not surprising, due to the difficulty of obtaining atrial capture with the pacing energies usually employed and the high rate of flutter waves that prevents the overdrive stimulation.

Apart from a single report[9] and other ones concerning only one or two occasional observations,[10-14] the other studies available have

Table 2.

	AF/AT	VT	SVRT	Stimulation	Success	Acceleration
Zoll (1985)	6	1		7	0	0
Rosenthal (1986)		1		O	1	0
Beaudry (1986)		1		U	1	0
Nauman (1986)		2		O	2	0
Barold (1987)		1		O	1	0
Luck (1987)		1	1	O	2	0
Luck (1988)		16		O	14	1
Klein (1988)		5		P	3	0
Estes (1989)		9		P/O	5	1
Estes (1989)		–	13	P/O	11	0
Grubb (1990)		7		O	7	1

Literature reports on termination of tachyarrhythmias by NTCP.
Numbers are referred to the patient's number, not to the tachycardia episodes treated.
AF = atrial flutter; AT = atrial tachycardia; VT = ventricular tachycardia;
SVRT = supraventricular reentrant tachycardia; U = underdrive; O = overdrive;
P = programmed.

tested the NTCP not on spontaneous arrhythmias but for the interruption of reentrant tachycardias induced by endocavitary stimulation in the electrophysiology laboratory.[15-17] Although these studies are important for assessing the safety and the efficacy of NTCP, the information available for the use of the technique in the clinical ground are necessarily limited, since the response of the spontaneous arrhythmias to the external stimulation can be different. On the contrary, our experience concerns the use of NTCP as first choice treatment of sustained spontaneous ventricular and supraventricular tachycardias. In our hands, NTCP was highly effective in terminating VT when overdrive pacing was possible, while the arrhythmia was interrupted in a lower percentage of the 14 patients when underdrive pacing was used. Actually, since the maximum pacing rate of our pacemaker was 160 ppm (80 ppm in the first device), overdrive pacing was not possible in all the cases with tachycardia rate over that value.

Nevertheless, it is known that VT with the highest rate are more difficult to interrupt by pacing techniques,[18] so that the lower success rate observed in patients with tachycardia rate more than 160 ppm might be due either to the lower efficacy of underdrive pacing or to the lower responsivity of the higher rate ventricular tachycardias to pacing. However, it can be supposed that with the availability of devices capable of higher pacing rates, the success rate of the technique might have been higher. This hypothesis is confirmed by the report of Grubb[9] who was able to terminate a total of 18 of 18 VT episodes by overdrive NTCP at a rate of 200 ppm. Actually, in a patient in whom intravenous propafenone reduced the tachycardia rate from 165 to 130 ppm, a previously unsuccessful burst at 160 ppm was able to interrupt the arrhythmia.

It has been recognized that increasing the current for endocardial burst facilitates capture and ventricular tachycardia termination.[19] Luck et al.[15] found that the external pacing threshold required for termination of VT was significantly higher than that required to pace the same patient in sinus rhythm. In our patients, we observed two cases in whom lower energies (60 and 70 mA), although capturing the ventricle, were repeatedly ineffective, while the same bursts at higher current (100 and 150 mA) were successful. It can be argued that higher energies may be able to, at the same time, depolarize a wider myocardial mass and enter even a partially protected reentrant circuit.

Supraventricular reentrant tachycardias seem more susceptible to be interrupted by NTCP than ventricular tachycardias. In fact, in SVT, not only the success rate was higher (71% vs 40%), but also the number of attempts necessary to terminate the arrhythmia in responders was lower. Often they were interrupted by a few stimuli at the first attempt. Even Estes[17] reports good results: out of 209 episodes of SVT as many as 168 (80%) were interrupted by a programmed single extrastimulus and another 28 (13%) by double extrastimuli.

The better results obtained in supraventricular tachycardias can be explained by the fact that all of them were reentrant arrhythmias and hence susceptible to be interrupted by pacing. In particular, although the limited number of our patients does not allow a statistical analysis, we obtained better results in atrioventricular than in intranodal reentrant tachycardias. It is conceivable that the success rate in this arrhythmia could be low because of the smaller reentrant circuit and the fact that neither the atrium nor the ventricle are part of the circuit itself. In fact, in atrioventricular tachycardia, ventricular capture itself can terminate the arrhythmia, while in intranodal tachycardia, the possibility of entering the circuit can be limited by lack of ventriculoatrial retroconduction or failure of atrial capture. The last eight cases of SVT have been treated at the first attempt with a maximum energy burst, because we observed that, by high transcutaneous energy, it can be possible to obtain atrial capture. The consequent possibility of achieving a simultaneous four chamber depolarization increases the likelihood of terminating the arrhythmia.

In 2 of the 36 patients (5.6%), NTCP produced worsening of the arrhythmia: a VT acceleration and an induction of ventricular fibrillation in a SVT complicating an acute myocardial infarction. Tachycardia acceleration has been observed in 3 of the 39 patients (13%) with VT treated by NTCP in the previous studies.[9,15,17] Indeed, there is a no reason to expect that NTCP could be devoid of a risk already well recognized with endocardial stimulation, where the incidence of ventricular tachycardia worsening ranges from 4% to 24%.[3,18,20] A substantial improvement for the technique would be the availability of pacing devices able to perform not only an underdrive or overdrive pacing, but also programmed stimulation. The feasibility of an external cardiac programmed stimulation has been already demonstrated.[16,17] The advantages are obvious:

1. It can reduce the pacing time and then the patient discomfort due to muscle and cutaneous nerve stimulation;
2. It minimizes the risk of tachycardia acceleration.

In fact, the endocardial synchronized extrastimuli technique, although less effective than multiple capture methods, has been reported to result in arrhythmia acceleration in less than 1% of the episodes, as compared with approximately 5% of arrhythmia worsening by multiple capture or burst technique.[20] So the possibility of gradually increasing the aggressiveness of the procedure, beginning with a single extrastimulus up to the burst, permits avoidance of unnecessary risk and discomfort to the patients responding to the initial part of the protocol.

In our experience, the tolerability of NTCP by the patients was acceptable since the stimulation attempts to interrupt the arrhythmia are all of short duration and the use of high energies is not necessarily limited by the tolerance of the patient, as happens when the technique is used for the treatment of bradyarrhythmias where longer pacing periods are required. Actually, the patient, once properly informed, can usually tolerate the discomfort of high energies pacing, if used for a few seconds. Thus, before considering an attempt ineffective, one should try the highest current the patient can tolerate.

Conclusion

NTCP can be regarded today as an effective method that joins the other means already available to the cardiologist for the interruption of hemodynamically stable ventricular and supraventricular reentrant tachycardias. While the great majority of supraventricular reentrant tachycardias are easily responsive to the technique, termination of ventricular tachycardias seems less predictable.

Its drawbacks include a suboptimal tolerance by some patients and the risk of arrhythmia worsening, mandating a defibrillatory unit to be always at hand.

A further clinical experience with new devices provided by higher pacing rates and programmed stimulation facilities is warranted and will complete our knowledge over the full potentiality of the NTCP.

References

1. Fischer JD, Mehra R, Furman S: Termination of ventricular tachycardia with bursts of rapid ventricular pacing. Am J Cardiol 41:94, 1978.
2. Gardner M, Waxman H, Buxton A, et al.: Termination of ventricular tachycardia: Evaluation of a new pacing method. Am J Cardiol 50:1338, 1982.
3. Saksena S, Chandran P, Shah Y, et al.: Comparative efficacy of transvenous cardioversion and pacing in patients with sustained ventricular tachycardia: A prospective randomized crossover study. Circulation 72:153, 1985.
4. Massumi RA, Kistin AD, Tawakkol AA: Termination of reciprocating tachycardia by atrial stimulation. Circulation 36:637, 1967.
5. Durrer D, Schoo L, Schuilemburg RM, et al.: The role of premature beats in the initiation and the termination of supraventricular tachycardia in the Wolf-Parkinson-White syndrome. Circulation 36:644, 1967.
6. Wellens HJ, Bar FW, Vanagt EL, et al.: The differentiation between ventricular tachycardia and supraventricular tachycardia with aberrant conduction: the value of the 12 lead electrocardiogram. *In:* What's New in Electrocardiography? Wellens HJ, Kulbertus HE (eds). Martinus Nijhoff Publishers, 1981, p. 184.
7. Farri J, Wellens HJ: The value of the electrocardiogram in diagnosing site of origin and mechanism of supraventricular tachycardia. *In:* What's new in electrocardiography? Wellens HJ, Kulbertus HE (eds). Martinus Nijhoff Publishers, 1981, p. 131.
8. Zoll PM, Zoll RH, Falk RH, et al.: External temporary cardiac pacing: clinical trials. Circulation 71:937, 1985.

9. Grubb BP, Temesy-Armos P, Hahn H, et al.: The clinical use of external noninvasive pacing in the termination of sustained ventricular tachycardia. PACE 13:1092, 1990.
10. Rosenthal M, Shamato N, Marchlinsky F, et al.: Noninvasive cardiac pacing for termination of sustained, uniform ventricular tachycardia. Am J Cardiol 58:561, 1986.
11. Beaudry PR, Rosengarten MD, Nadeau L: Termination of ventricular tachycardia with transcutaneous cardiac pacing. Can Med Assoc J 134:145, 1986.
12. Nauman D'Alnoncourt C, Becht I, Haase HJ, et al.: Transcutaneous cardiac noninvasive pacing. Herzschrittmacher 6:5, 1986.
13. Barold SS, Falkoff MD, Ong LS, et al.: Termination of ventricular tachycardia by transcutaneous cardiac pacing. Am Heart J 114:180, 1987.
14. Luck JC, Davis D: Termination of sustained tachycardia by external noninvasive pacing. PACE 10:1125, 1987.
15. Luck JC, Grubb BP, Artman SE, et al.: Termination of sustained ventricular tachycardia by external noninvasive pacing. Am J Cardiol 61:574, 1988.
16. Klein LS, Miles WM, Heger JJ, et al.: Transcutaneous pacing: Patient tolerance, strength-interval relations and feasibility for programmed electrical stimulation. Am J Cardiol 62:1126, 1988.
17. Estes NAM III, Deering TF, Manolis AS, et al.: External programmed stimulation for noninvasive termination of sustained supraventricular and ventricular tachycardia. J Am Coll Cardiol 63:177, 1989.
18. Fischer JD, Matos JA, Kim SG: Antitachycardia pacing and stimulation. *In*: Tachycardias: Mechanisms, diagnosis, treatment. Josephson ME, Wellens HJ (eds). Lea and Febiger, Philadelphia, 1984, p. 413.
19. Waxman H, Cain M, Greenspan A, et al.: Termination of ventricular tachycardia with ventricular stimulation: Salutary effects of increased current strength. Circulation 65:800, 1982.
20. Fischer JD, Kim SG, Matos JA, et al.: Comparative effectiveness of pacing techniques of well tolerated sustained ventricular tachycardia. PACE 6:915, 1983.

Chapter 11

Noninvasive Cardiac Pacing for Ventricular Tachycardia: Feasibility of Electrophysiological Testing

Jerry C. Luck, MD, Michael L. Markel, MD

Zoll introduced noninvasive external (or transcutaneous) cardiac pacing in 1952 for patients suffering from Stokes-Adams syncope.[1] The concept and the method were valid so the initial clinical attempts to prevent syncope and death from ventricular asystole proved successful.[2,3] In 1956, Zoll et al.[4] published animal experiments on external pacing and the induction of ventricular tachycardia (VT) and fibrillation and supraventricular tachycardia (SVT). In the dog, rapid external pacing at rates between 500 and 1200 ppm did not induce ventricular tachycardia. However, if rapid and prolonged pacing produced hypotension, then some dogs did develop ventricular and atrial fibrillation. In their pigs made ischemic by ligation of the circumflex artery, burst external pacing could easily induce ventricular tachycardia and fibrillation. They also observed that atrial fibrillation and an atrioventricular (AV) nodal tachycardia were induced in their ischemic pig model.[4] In 1960, Zoll et al.[5] were able to demonstrate that external pacing at normal heart rates could prevent recurrences of VT in some patients with severe bradycardia from AV block. However, external pacing was painful, so this simple, rapid, and safe

From *Noninvasive Transcutaneous Cardiac Pacing* edited by Pierre Birkui, M.D., Jacques Trigano, M.D., and Paul Zoll, M.D., © 1993, Futura Publishing Company, Inc., Mount Kisco, NY.

technique was replaced by the transvenous endocardial pacing method around 1960.[6,7]

Endocardial cardiac stimulation techniques were applied in the early 1970s to induce and terminate sustained VT and paroxysmal supraventricular tachycardia (PSVT).[8-10] In individuals with sustained monomorphic VT and coronary disease, programmed ventricular extrastimuli and burst ventricular pacing are able to induce VT in 85%-95% of cases.[11] Single and multiple ventricular stimuli have been shown to terminate 60%-90% of induced episodes of sustained monomorphic VT in the clinical electrophysiology laboratory.[12,13] Similarly, programmed atrial extrastimuli are used to induce PSVT. The endocardial stimulation and recording method has several advantages. Pacing can be performed from any cardiac chamber and recordings can be obtained from multiple sites. Thus, it facilitates making a precise diagnosis and mapping of a reentrant tachycardia circuit. Although not without risk, the transvenous endocardial pacing method is relatively painless. Permanent transvenous pacing is now available with sophisticated antitachycardia algorithms to interrupt paroxysmal VT and PSVT.[14] Despite these advances in antitachycardia pacing, the clinician continues to need a rapid and safe technique for the emergency termination of sustained VT and PSVT without having to resort to direct current cardioversion. Thus, interest in external pacing, or noninvasive transcutaneous cardiac pacing (NTCP), has resurfaced and this method may play an increasing role in antitachycardia pacing. Our aim is to determine if this is feasible.

Clinical Reports and Trials

Ventricular tachycardia: There are several case reports of external pacing to terminate a sustained monomorphic VT.[15-17] They used either underdrive or overdrive pacing with a standard commercially available device. The initial clinical trial compared the effectiveness of external pacing to endocardial ventricular pacing for termination of VT.[18] In 14 patients, there were 16 VT morphologies that could be reproducibly terminated in the electrophysiology laboratory with endocardial overdrive right ventricular pacing. Thirteen of these patients had a previous myocardial infarction and one patient without coronary disease had a dilated cardiomyopathy. The endocardial method used synchronized burst of 3-9 beats at 2 times diastolic threshold, while the external method used asynchronous burst pacing initially at 20 mA above pacing threshold. The average cycle length of sustained VT was 392 ± 97 msec (range: 690 to 300 msec). Fourteen of the 16 trials were performed on an antiarrhythmic agent which slowed the VT. External pacing terminated 14 of 16 (88%) sustained VT morphologies. The external pacing threshold current in sinus rhythm was 76 ± 14 mA. It was difficult to consistently capture the heart at 20 mA above threshold during VT. The pacing current needed to consistently capture and terminate VT averaged 107 ± 23 mA (range: 60 to 140 mA). The external burst pacing cycle length used to terminate VT averaged 282 ± 44 msec and was similar to the endocardial cycle length (298 ± 93 msec) used to terminate VT. External pacing failed to terminate a slow VT (690 msec) in a patient on amiodarone and mexiletine who had previously undergone a median sternotomy for coronary bypass surgery. It accelerated VT in another patient. However, external pacing compared favorably to the gold standard endocardial pacing for the termination of VT. This study seemed to indicate that external pacing might be useful for follow-up or serial drug testing in patients with sustained VT.

In contrast to our results, Estes et al.[19] could terminate VT with external pacing in only 5 of 14 (36%) episodes induced in the laboratory. The methodology was different. They attempted to terminate VT with external pacing using threshold values or at 30 mA above threshold. At threshold, it is unlikely that closely coupled extrastimuli were achieved. Likewise, rapid external pacing near threshold (mean 72 mA) probably fails to consistently capture the ventricle. Altamura et al.[20,21] have terminated sustained VT with external pacing in 6 of 14 (43%) and 8 of 20 (40%) episodes. They were limited by a device that has an upper pacing rate of 160 ppm. The rate of VT averaged 177 ppm.[20] The pacing current needed to terminate VT was 106 ± 29 mA.[21] Grubb et al.[22] used external pacing to successfully terminate 18 of 18 episodes of sustained VT in seven patients. The VT rates were slow at an average of 146 ppm. External overdrive pacing was performed at 200 ppm and at 120 mA. The mixed results on efficacy of termination of VT is more a function of technical limitations and not a failure of the method. Observations from these four authors suggest that external pacing can be used effectively to terminate sustained monomorphic VT (Fig. 1). However, all authors did see acceleration of sustained VT with external pacing. All hinted at external pacing being uncomfortable, and the thresholds needed to terminate VT are generally greater than 100 mA.

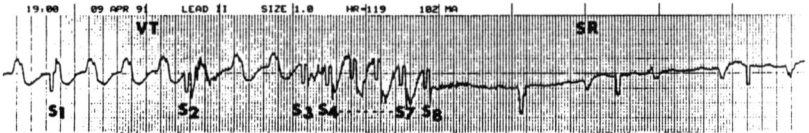

Figure 1. *Termination of ventricular tachycardia (VT) with external pacing. There is a spontaneous sustained VT at a rate of 120 ppm in a patient taking amiodarone. A Zoll PD (combination pacer-defibrillator) is set at a pacing rate of 180 ppm. The 4:1 pacing mode button is depressed. The initial current output is 0 mA, thus the initial stimuli (S_1 and S_2) do not capture. The current output is abruptly increased to 102 mA and the third stimulus (S_3) fuses with a VT complex. The 4:1 button is released and stimuli are delivered at 180 ppm for 6 stimuli (S_3-S_8). At S_8, the 4:1 button is again depressed and the output returned to 0 mA. There is resumption of sinus rhythm (SR) after overdrive pacing for 4 beats (S_4-S_7).*

There are only incidental reports of external pacing being used to induce sustained VT. The first clinical induction of sustained VT was reported by Zoll et al.[23] in 1985. In this single example, external pacing was used to test antiarrhythmic efficacy. Klein et al.[24] induced VT in three of five patients with sustained monomorphic VT. They indicated that external stimulation for induction of VT was theoretically feasible but would be limited to a small patient population with low pacing thresholds. In our laboratory, we have successfully induced sustained VT with external pacing in seven patients. The external pacing sequences used for induction were the same used for endocardial stimulation in three patients. In three other patients, additional extrastimuli were needed to induce VT. In one patient, VT was easier to induce with NTCP (Table 1). Larger trials are needed to determine the efficacy of external pacing for induction of VT (Fig. 1).

Electrophysiological Considerations for Induction of Tachycardia

The induction of sustained monomorphic VT in patients remote from myocardial infarction is generally secondary to reentry. Thus, the appropriate circuit with an area of slow conduction and unidirectional block is necessary. In the laboratory, induction of VT is dependent on critically timed extrastimuli to initiate the tachycardia.[9,10] Introducing the extrastimuli at a site close to the reentrant loop favors

Table 1. Induction of Ventricular Tachycardia

Pt.	Age/Sex	VT Morph	VT CL	VT Rate	ENDO Induction	EXP Induction	EXP-mA Threshold/ Induction
1	46/M	RBBB/NW	500	120	500(280)	500(280)	70/120
2	58/M	RBBB/LA	470	127	500(360)	500(360)	125/140
3	78/F	RBBB/NW	340	176	500(260, 270)	500(260, 270)	65/120
4	56/M	RBBB/NW	440	193	500(290, 240)	500(240)	70/120
5	77/M	RBBB/LA	320	187	500(280, 230)	500(300, 280, 270)	105/140
6	72/M	LBBB/LA	280	214	400(230)	400(222, 220, 200)	70/120
7	73/F	RBBB/RA	280	214	500(230, 210, 200)	500(230, 220, 280)	80/140

ENDO = endocardial pacing; EXP = external pacing; EXP-mA = external pacing stimulus amplitude; LBBB = left bundle branch block; RBBB = right bundle branch block; LA = left axis; NW = northwest or extreme right axis; RA = right axis; VT = ventricular tachycardia; VT/CL = ventricular tachycardia cycle length; VT Morph = ventricular tachycardia QRS morphology. Note: The stimulus drive trains of either 500 or 400 msec and extrastimuli are in parentheses. (S2, S3, S4) indicates triple extrastimuli.

induction of VT. With the endocardial stimulation method, multiple sites can be used.

Our observations suggest that external pacing can introduce critically timed extrastimuli for induction of VT.[25] Effective and functional refractory periods (ERP, FRP) were obtained in 17 patients with both the endocardial and external pacing methods. At twice threshold, endocardial ERP was 235 ± 32 msec and FRP was 262 ± 29 msec. The external pacing ERP values were: 276 ± 29 msec at 10 mA above threshold, 254 ± 32 msec at 1.5 times threshold, and 237 ± 39 msec at twice threshold. External pacing ERP at threshold plus 10 mA and at 1.5 times threshold were significantly greater than endocardial ERP at twice threshold. However, external cardiac pacing ERP at twice threshold was similar to endocardial ERP at twice threshold (237 ± 39 msec vs 235 ± 32 msec).

External pacing ERP values at twice threshold were equal to or less than endocardial values in 7 of 17 patients. In an additional 10 patients, the external pacing ERP values at twice threshold were greater than endocardial ones. However, the margin of difference was less than 30 msec in all but two. At twice threshold, external pacing FRP was significantly longer than endocardial FRP (262 ± 29 vs 280 ± 29 msec, $p \leq 0.005$). The significant difference in FRP values probably reflects the method of measurement since external pacing frequently obscures the electrogram of conventional monitors. It is realistic to assume that external pacing can achieve closely coupled extrastimuli that are necessary to induce ventricular tachycardia. The external pacing threshold in sinus rhythm averaged 64 ± 14 mA and at twice threshold averaged 128 mA. The major limitation of using external pacing at these current amplitudes is the severe skeletal muscle discomfort.

Current strength-interval curves were constructed with both external and endocardial pacing methods in these same 17 patients.[25] The external pacing data were obtained at a pulse width of 40 msec and slightly above threshold (range: 40 to 80 mA). Initially, endocardial currents were applied at 2 msec pulse width and at twice threshold (range: 0.2 to 1 mA). Thus, only the shapes of the curves were compared at ERP. The curves were parallel in 14 patients and nonparallel in 3 patients. In the parallel group, the curves were superimposed in 5 patients but displaced significantly to the right in 9 patients (Fig. 2). In the 3 patients with nonparallel curves, the external curve was sloping. We assume that external pacing initially

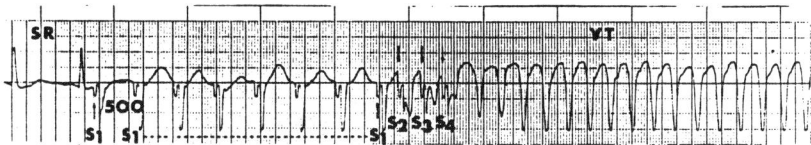

Figure 2. *Induction of ventricular tachycardia (VT) with an external pacer that is triggered by a standard programmable stimulator. Sustained monomorphic VT is induced using a typical ventricular drive train of 8 stimuli (S_1) at 500 msec and programmed extrastimuli (S_2 220, S_3 220, S_4 200 msec). The induced VT cycle length is 280 msec. SR = sinus rhythm.*

activates the epicardial surface. Then, the differences in endocardial and external parallel but shifted curves reflect markedly disparate initial sites of activation. In the nonparallel group, the different curves may simply reflect the current outputs used for the two methods. The endocardial curves were constructed at 2–20 times threshold while external pacing curves were from data using threshold to 140 mA (just over twice threshold). The conclusions drawn from these observations were that external pacing refractoriness is very similar to endocardial refractoriness and theoretically should be comparable for the induction and termination of VT with critically timed extrastimuli.

Can external pacing introduce ventricular extrastimuli at multiple sites? In a preliminary report, Markel et al.[26] have examined ventricular activation patterns during external pacing. In 16 patients, the external pacing electrodes location on the thorax were varied and the endocardial activation sequences analyzed. The surface QRS complexes were recorded in leads 1, 2, and 3 at each of the 5 pacing sites. The threshold current was analyzed at each site. External pacing threshold current varied considerably when the transcutaneous electrode positions were changed. In general, threshold current was less when the cathodal patch was near the point of maximum impulse (88 ± 24 mA) or along the upper sternal border (100 ± 28 mA). If the electrodes are reversed such that the cathode is positioned on the back, then the threshold increases to 133 ± 17 mA. When both patches were on the anterior chest (right anterior to apical cathode), the threshold averaged 107 ± 29 mA. When pacing at a fifth site on the left anterior chest (cathode) to a left posterior (anode), the threshold was 133 ± 17 mA. The data on stable ventricular capture varied tremendously with changing the electrode position. Capture was consistent when the cathode was at the apex (15 of 16 patients) or at the left upper sternal border (14 of 16 patients). When both electrodes were on the anterior chest, there was consistent capture in 11 of 16 patients. At the two remaining sites, ventricular capture was generally inconsistent or absent. When the cathode was placed on the back and the anode anteriorly, consistent capture was present in only 2 of 16 patients. When the cathode was at the left anterior chest position and the anode posterior, consistent capture was seen in only 5 patients.

Markel et al.[26] observed that the earliest site of ventricular activation was different with different electrode positions. When the cathode electrode was positioned at the point of maximum impulse (apex) and the anode posterior, the right ventricular apex was activated initially in 13 of 15 patients. Upon moving the cathodal electrode to the left sternal border, the initial activation site shifts to the anterior and basal right ventricle (nearer the right ventricular outflow tract) in 14 patients. If the cathodal patch remains at the apex and the anodal patch is moved to the right upper chest, then the left ventricle is frequently activated initially (9 of 15 patients). At this same electrodes position, the right ventricular apex is activated in 6 of 15 patients. At the two remaining sites where capture was frequently inconsistent, the earliest site of activation varied from either the right or left ventricles. As is seen with the endocardial pacing method, the ventricular pacing site can be varied with external pacing (Fig. 3). When using different transcutaneous electrode positions, external pacing could be used to perform programmed stimulation from multiple ventricular pacing sites.

If the surface electrocardiogram is analyzed in the standard leads at each electrode position change, then certain patterns become apparent. It follows that right ventricular apical pacing produces a predominantly upright QRS complex in lead 1 with a negative complex in leads 2 and 3. Pacing along the upper left sternal border tends to produce a different pattern with lead 1 positive; lead 2 positive; and lead 3 positive, negative, or biphasic. When the left ventricle is activated, lead 1 is negative. The surface electrocardiogram pattern reflects the change in electrode position with external pacing.

Presently, there are some technical limitations which will need to be overcome before general clinical use can proceed. The problem of external pacing discomfort remains. At most positions, the average threshold current needed for pacing was greater than 90 mA. At some

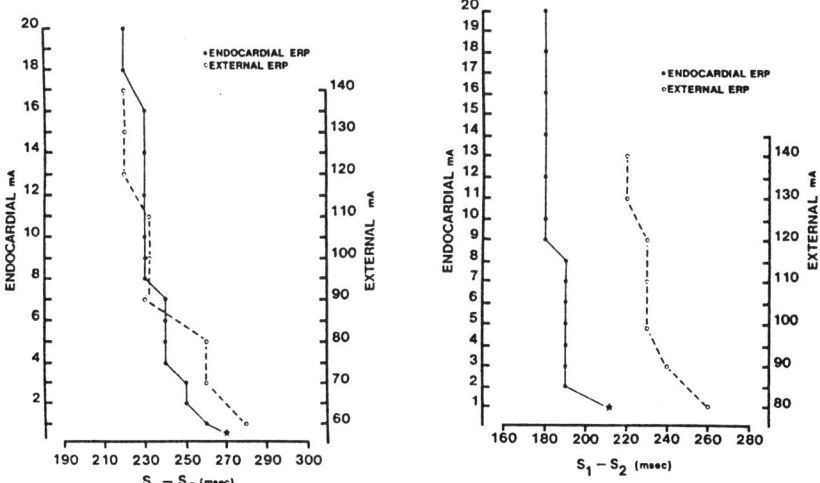

Figure 3. *Comparison of current strength-effective refractory period (ERP) for external and endocardial pacing. Coupling intervals (S_1-S_2 msec) are on the X axis. On the Y axis, endocardial current (mA) is on the left and external current (mA) is on the right. The left panel shows both curves are parallel and superimposed at comparable ERP values. The right panel shows parallel curves but the external one is significantly shifted to the right. The * represents ERP at endocardial twice threshold. The initial external pacing ERP was obtained at threshold plus 10 mA. Reproduced with permission from Luck et al.[25]*

of the positions, capture was inconsistent and at best intermittent even at 140 mA. Thus, studies will need to be performed with moderate sedation as was the case in the study by Markel et al.[26] Likewise, the stability of the pacing position is not always consistent. In some cases, the electrodes' positions are constant but the electrocardiogram patterns and the activation sequences are changing. This is best explained by the fact that the heart's position in the thorax is not fixed and varies with position and respiration. Thus, the point of earliest activation changes because the area of myocardium closest to the fixed cathode is changing. The present devices have limitations on current amplitude. For ventricular tachycardia termination and induction, the current amplitudes may need to be twice threshold to achieve closely coupled intervals. This may be difficult since present devices have limits of 140 to 150 mA.

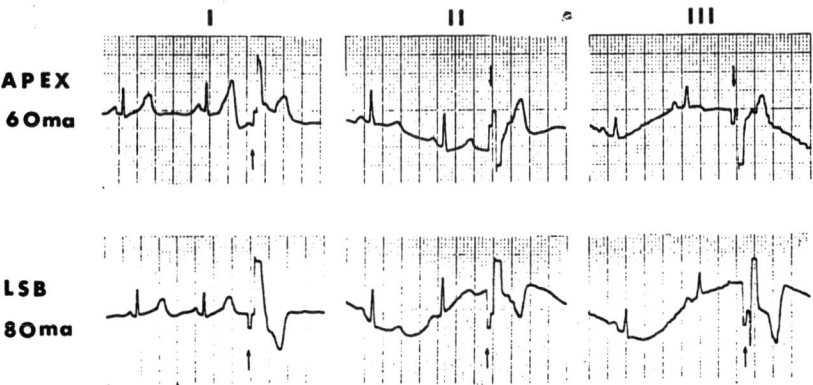

Figure 4. Depicts QRS configuration when the cathodal anterior electrode is shifted from the point of maximum impulse (APEX) to the upper left sternal border (LSB) for external pacing. The pacing threshold is listed for each site. Only surface leads 1, 2, and 3 are available and each shows two sinus complexes and a ventricular 7 complex generated by external pacing (at arrow). The QRS configuration of the paced beats designated APEX show a polarity that suggest right ventricular (RV) apical pacing (1, positive; 2 and 3, negative). The panel labeled LSB shows a different QRS morphology with leads 1, 2, and 3 depicting a positive complex. This pacing site is initially activating the RV out flow tract. Thus, different sites are activated by moving the anterior electrode. Note: the external stimulus artifact is 40 msec and there is another 40 msec blanking period before the QRS complex is seen.

Conclusion

Endocardial pacing techniques are useful for analyzing the mechanism of both supraventricular and ventricular tachycardias.[9] Pacing is frequently used to induce and terminate reentrant tachycardias. Serial testing of antiarrhythmic agents is one approach to treatment of sustained ventricular tachycardia. The present question is whether NTCP can be used to perform these functions. To date, external pacing has been used to terminate sustained ventricular tachycardia and may be nearly as effective as the endocardial method. Although not analyzed here, external pacing can terminate some sustained supraventricular tachycardias.[21] It is effective at interrupting AV reciprocating tachycardia and some AV nodal reentrant tachycardias because the ventricular stimuli have direct access to the reentrant loop. Whether or not external pacing should be routinely used for termination of supraventricular tachycardia, because of the potential induction of ventricular fibrillation, remains controversial. At present, external pacing rarely captures the atrium in humans but can provide closely coupled ventricular extrastimuli to induce ventricular tachycardia. At present, there are limited reports on induction of ventricular tachycardia. Finally, external pacing can stimulate multiple ventricular sites. If the limitations can be overcome, then external pacing could be used for serial drug testing after an initial invasive study.

References

1. Zoll PM: Resuscitation of the heart in ventricular standstill by external electric stimulation. N Engl J Med 247:768, 1952.
2. Zoll PM, Linenthal AJ, Norman LR, et al.: Treatment of Stokes-Adams disease by external electric stimulation of the heart. Circulation 9:482, 1954.
3. Zoll PM, Linenthal AJ, Norman LR, et al.: External electric stimulation of the heart in cardiac arrest. Arch Intern Med 96:639, 1955.
4. Zoll PM, Zoll RH, Linenthal AJ, et al.: The effects of external electric currents on the heart. Control of cardiac rhythm and induction and termination of cardiac arrhythmias. Circulation 14:745, 1956.
5. Zoll PM, Linenthal AJ, Zarsky LRN: Ventricular fibrillation. Treatment and prevention by external electric currents. N Engl J Med 262:105, 1960.
6. Furman S, Robinson G: Use of intracardiac pacemaker in correction of total heart block. Surg Forum 9:245, 1958.
7. Furman S, Schwedel JB: An intracardiac pacemaker for Stokes-Adams seizures. N Engl J Med 261:943, 1959.
8. Durrer D, Schoo L, Schuilenburg RM, et al.: The role of premature beats in the initiation and termination of supraventricular tachycardia in the Wolf-Parkinson-White syndrome. Circulation 34:644, 1967.
9. Wellens HJ: Value, limitations of programmed electrical stimulation of the heart in the study and treatment of tachycardias. Circulation 57:845, 1978.
10. Josephson ME, Horowitz LN: Electrophysiologic approach to therapy of recurrent sustained ventricular tachycardia. Am J Cardiol 43:631, 1979.
11. Buxton AE, Waxman HL, Marchlinski FE, et al.: Role of triple extrastimuli during electrophysiologic study of patients with documented sustained ventricular tachyarrhythmias. Circulation 69:532, 1984.
12. Fisher JD, Kim SG, Matos JA, et al.: Comparative effectiveness of pacing techniques of well tolerated sustained ventricular tachycardia. PACE 6:915, 1983.
13. Saksena S, Chandra P, Shah Y, et al.: Comparative efficacy of transvenous cardioversion and pacing in patients with sustained ventricular tachycardia: A prospective randomized crossover study. Circulation 72:153, 1985.

14. den Dulk K, Kersschot IE, Brugada P, et al.: Is there a universal antitachycardia pacing mode? Am J Cardiol 57:950, 1986.
15. Beaudry PR, Rosengarten MD, Nadeau Lo: Termination of ventricular tachycardia with transcutaneous cardiac pacing. Canadian Med Asso J 134:145, 1986.
16. Rosenthal ME, Stamato NJ, Marchlinski FE, et al.: Noninvasive cardiac pacing for termination of sustained uniformed ventricular tachycardia. Am J Cardiol 58:561, 1986.
17. Barold SS, Falkoff MD, Ong LS, et al.: Termination of ventricular tachycardia by transcutaneous cardiac pacing. Am Heart J 114:180, 1987.
18. Luck JC, Grubb BP, Artman SE, et al.: Termination of sustained ventricular tachycardia by external noninvasive pacing. Am J Cardiol 61:574, 1988.
19. Estes NAM III, Deering TF, Manolis AS, et al.: External cardiac programmed stimulation for noninvasive termination of sustained supraventricular and ventricular tachycardia. Am J Cardiol 63:177, 1989.
20. Altamura G, Bianconi L, Boccadamo R, et al.: Treatment of ventricular and supraventricular tachyarrhythmias by transcutaneous cardiac pacing. PACE 12:331, 1989.
21. Altamura G, Bianconi L, Toscano S, et al.: Transcutaneous cardiac pacing for termination of tachyarrhythmias. PACE 13:2026, 1990.
22. Grubb BP, Temesy-Armos P, Hahn H, et al.: The clinical use of external noninvasive pacing in the termination of sustained ventricular tachycardia. PACE 13:1092, 1990.
23. Zoll PM, Zoll RH, Falk RH, et al.: External noninvasive temporary cardiac pacing: Clinical trials. Circulation 71:937, 1985.
24. Klein LS, Miles WM, Heger JJ, et al.: Transcutaneous pacing: Patient tolerance, strength-interval relations and feasibility for programmed electrical stimulation. Am J Cardiol 62:1126, 1988.
25. Luck JC, Grubb BP, Markel ML: Description of the strength-interval relation with external noninvasive pacing. PACE 13:2031, 1990.
26. Markel ML, Grubb BP, Artman SE, et al.: The effect of external electrode location on endocardial activation and threshold during external pacing: Implications for programmed stimulation (abstr). RBM 12:87, 1990.

Chapter 12

Noninvasive Transcutaneous Cardiac Pacing for Termination of Sustained Supraventricular and Ventricular Tachycardias

N.A. Mark Estes III, MD, Thomas F. Deering, MD,
Antonis S. Manolis, MD, Deeb Salem, MD,
Paul M. Zoll, MD

Programmed electrical stimulation of the heart with the use of endocardial or epicardial pacing electrodes has been safely and effectively employed to terminate sustained supraventricular tachycardia (SVT) and ventricular tachycardia (VT).[1-5] Transcutaneous cardiac stimulation has become a standard tool for the temporary treatment of bradycardias.[6-8] Several investigators have used transcutaneous cardiac pacing to overdrive reentrant supraventricular and ventricular arrhythmias.[9-13] This promising technique has attracted attention because of its potential applications for the acute treatment of patients with cardiac tachyarrhythmic episodes. However, the conventional external pacemaker operates only in the demand mode within limited pacing rates, and thus underdrive or overdrive pacing for tachycardia termination is not feasible with the current device when the tachycardia rate is above its upper rate limit. Also, the present device does not have the capability of scanning by

From *Noninvasive Transcutaneous Cardiac Pacing* edited by Pierre Birkui, M.D., Jacques Trigano, M.D., and Paul Zoll, M.D., © 1993, Futura Publishing Company, Inc., Mount Kisco, NY.

delivering programmed synchronized extrastimuli, a safer pacing technique that can avoid tachycardia acceleration or degeneration to fibrillation.[4-14]

Because of these limitations of the conventional noninvasive external pacemakers, we developed a noninvasive temporary pacing system that can track the output of a standard programmable cardiac stimulator and allow synchronized scanning of diastole with extrastimuli and overdrive pacing and previously reported on the results with this device.[15] With this system, a standard termination protocol, using single or double extrastimuli, as well as bursts of synchronous overdrive pacing, was employed and its efficacy, safety, and tolerance was tested in 223 separate tachycardias in 22 patients.

Methods

Noninvasive Transcutaneous Cardiac Programmed Stimulation

The conventional transcutaneous external temporary pacemaker (Zoll NTP, ZMI Corporation, Cambridge, MA) modified for this study consisted of a cardiac monitor, three-lead electrocardiographic recorder, and transcutaneous pacemaker capable of demand pacing via self-adhesive high impedance pads.[6-8] For bradycardia pacing, it functions in demand mode by sensing surface QRS voltage changes of appropriate amplitude and slow rate. Pacing is accomplished via the external electrodes (pads) placed anteriorly at the cardiac apex or on the left parasternal border, and posteriorly between the left scapula and spine. The pacing stimuli have a pulse duration (width) of 40 msec and a constant current rectilinear design and can be delivered at rates up to 180 ppm and amplitudes up to 140 mA. Appropriate filtering reduces the distortion of the electrocardiogram from the large stimulus current and thus facilitates interpretation of the monitor recordings of the surface leads during pacing.

This standard noninvasive transcutaneous temporary pacemaker was modified to track the output of a programmable cardiac stimulator for the purpose of delivering synchronized extrastimuli and overdrive rapid pacing during a tachycardia. A synchronization signal coinciding with each sensed QRS complex was sent to the programmable cardiac stimulator via an output circuit added to the external pacemaker. The stimulator was then used to trigger the pacemaker to deliver synchronized extrastimuli and rapid pacing at programmable coupling intervals and rates. Furthermore, the electrocardiographic monitor of the transcutaneous pacemaker was relayed to a physiological recorder. On the oscilloscope of this recorder two surface electrocardiographic leads and up to four intracardiac recordings filtered at 30–500 Hz were displayed. A 14-channel tape recorder was employed to store all recordings for subsequent playback and analysis. The posterior R-2 pad (R-2 Corporation, Skokie, IL) was in place throughout the study, while the apical pad was ready for immediate positioning in case there was need for cardioversion or defibrillation.

Pacing Protocol

Prior to attempting induction of the tachyarrhythmia, the ventricular capture threshold by external pacing was determined by gradually increasing the current output of the transcutaneous pacemaker to the point of consistent ventricular capture during the patient's native rhythm. With effective ventricular capture that could be obtained at 5 mA or up to maximum 30 mA over this capture threshold, pacing with external cardiac programmed stimulation was performed during an episode of a hemodynamically stable sustained tachycardia. The initial stage of the pacing protocol for arrhythmia termination consisted of scanning diastole with a single extrastimulus by 10–20 msec decrements to the effective refractory period of the ventricle. Subsequently, the first extrastimulus was placed 10 msec beyond the refractory period and a second extrastimulus was scanned by 10–20 msec decrements from late diastole to the effective refractory period. If the two extrastimuli did not result in arrhythmia termination, then at least three bursts of rapid overdrive pacing were used at 10 to 50 ppm faster than the tachycardia rate. It took approximately 60 seconds to complete the protocol with single and double extrastimuli followed by burst pacing. An unsuccessful attempt was defined as completion of single and double extrastimuli and at least three bursts of rapid pacing without termination of the arrhythmia.

Endocardial pacing, and in one case cardioversion, was used for tachycardia termination, when the external pacing failed to terminate the arrhythmia. In three patients, tachycardia terminations with external cardiac programmed stimulation were attempted over the course of serial electropharmacological testing and thus data from multiple days are reported. Discomfort was rated by the patient on a scale 1 to 4 during and after the procedure and was characterized as mild (1), moderate (2), severe (3), or intolerable (4). If needed, sedation with up to 7.5 mg of intravenous diazepam was used.

Results

Study Patients and Clinical Data

Table 1 describes the overall results. Selection of study patients was based on previous episodes of hemodynamically tolerated spontaneous SVT (13 patients) or VT (9 patients). The study protocol had been approved by the Human Investigations Review Committee of our medical center and a written informed consent was obtained from each patient. The study included 22 patients, 5 women and 17 men, with an average age of 54 ± 15 years (range: 28 to 72). The arrhythmia was SVT in 13 patients, 10 of whom had Wolff-Parkinson-White syndrome, with 9 having only orthodromic atrioventricular reciprocating tachycardias, and 1 both orthodromic and antidromic reciprocating tachycardia. Three patients had dual atrioventricular nodal pathways with atrioventricular nodal reentrant tachycardia. Sustained monomorphic ventricular tachycardia was the arrhythmia in 9 patients. All these 9 patients had coronary artery disease as the underlying structural heart disease and 8 of them had a history of previous myocardial infarction. The left ventricular ejection fraction of the patients with ventricular tachycardia averaged $31 \pm 14\%$.

Noninvasive transcutaneous pacing with programmed stimulation was studied in 209 episodes of SVT in 13 patients. Of the 13 patients with SVT, only 4 patients with reciprocating tachycardia in the setting of Wolff-Parkinson-White syndrome were receiving drugs with antiarrhythmic activity including flecainide (2 patients), encainide (1 patient), and propafenone (1 patient). External pacing was attempted in the emergency room in 1 patient presenting with spontaneous orthodromic reciprocating tachycardia. Among the other patients with SVT, before external pacing was attempted, 11 had the tachycardia induced during a diagnostic electrophysiology study, while in one patient atrioventricular nodal reentry tachycardia was noninvasively induced reproducibly with the use of an implanted antitachycardia pacemaker.

A total of 14 episodes of VT were studied using external programmed stimulation in 9 patients undergoing intracardiac electrophysiology studies. Ten of these 14 episodes were induced while the patients were receiving antiarrhythmic agents. One additional patient with large left pleural effusion was excluded from the study because ventricular capture could not be affected by external pacing with up to 120 mA.

Supraventricular Tachycardias

A total of 20 episodes of atrioventricular nodal reentrant tachycardia were studied in three patients. Noninvasive transcutaneous cardiac programmed stimulation was successful in all 16 attempts in one patient, all three attempts in a second patient, and none of three attempts in a third patient. The arrhythmia could be reproducibly terminated with endocardial programmed ventricular stimulation in both patients in whom the transcutaneous technique was successful. In the patient in whom external pacing was unsuccessful despite effective ventricular capture, the tachycardia could not be reliably terminated with endocardial ventricular stimulation, although it was terminated with endocardial atrial pacing.

In Figure 1 (panels A-D) selected rhythm strips of four distinct episodes of SVT from patient 1 are shown. Atrioventricular nodal reentrant tachycardia had been documented by standard criteria as the mechanism of the SVT (previous electrophysiological study). A permanent scanning antitachycardia pacemaker (PASAR, Telectronics Corp., Sydney, Australia) had been implanted for this drug-refractory arrhythmia with the endocardial electrode positioned in the right atrial appendage and used for arrhythmia detection and termination. By programming the antitachycardia pacemaker to deliver a single extrastimulus, the SVT was reproducibly induced (16 times). One episode of this noninvasive initiation of the SVT with a single endocardial extrastimulus from the pacemaker coupled-in 280 msec after a sensed P wave in sinus rhythm is shown in panel A. In panel B, the tachycardia is terminated by the modified external pacemaker with a single extrastimulus. Double extrastimuli in C and rapid pacing in D are also successful in terminating the tachycardia. In another

Table 1. Results and Patient Characteristics

Pt.	Age, Sex	Heart Disease	Arrhythmia	CL (msec)	Drugs	Episodes of Tachycardia	Total ECPS	Successful ECPS	Threshold in mA	Discomfort*
1	36, F	ASD repair	AVNRT	360	—	16	16	16	40	1
2	52, M	CAD	AVNRT	390	—	1	3	0	70	3
3	72, M	NSHD	AVNRT	450	—	3	3	3	65	3
4	50, M	WPW	AVRT	330	Propafenone	1	6	0	40	2
5	22, M	WPW	AVRT	350	—	5	5	3	90	1
6	57, M	WPW, MVP	AVRT	345	—	5	5	4	65	2
7	72, M	WPW	AVRT	290	—	5	5	4	78	2
8	68, M	WPW	AVRT	640	Flecainide	60	60	58	40	1
9	28, F	WPW	AVRT	460	Flecainide	100	100	98	68	2
10	40, M	WPW	AVRT	360	—	2	2	4	70	3
11	32, M	WPW	AVRT	290	—	5	5	2	75	2
12	34, F	WPW	AVRT	450	Flecainide	2	2	2	80	3
13	54, F	WPW	AVRT	360	Pirmenol	4	4	4	65	4
14	67, F	CAD	VT	340	Flecainide	1	2	0	90	4
				440	Flecainide	1	2	0	87	3
				420	Encainide	1	2	1	90	2

Sustained Supraventricular and Ventricular Tachycardias

	Age, Sex	Disease		CL	Drug				
15	70, M	CAD	VT	440	Amiodarone	1	1	1	2
				300	Amiodarone & procainamide	1	1	1	2
16	56, M	CAD	VT	450	Flecainide	1	2	0	3
				320	—	1	1	1	1
17	68, M	CAD	VT	360	Flecainide	1	1	0	3
18	58, M	CAD	VT	270	—	1	1	0	2
19	55, M	CAD	VT	380	—	1	4	0	3
20	60, M	CAD	VT	350	—	1	3	0	3
				340	Procainamide & mexiletine	1	1	0	3
21	67, M	CAD	VT	390	Tocainide & quinidine	1	3	0	3
22	62, M	CAD	VT	450	Amiodarone & mexiletine	1	1	1	2

*Discomfort: 1 = mild, 2 = moderate, 3 = severe, 4 = intolerable; ASD = atrial septal defect; AVNRT = atrioventricular nodal reentrant tachycardia; AVRT = atrioventricular reciprocating tachycardia; CAD = coronary artery disease; ECPS = external cardiac programmed stimulation; NSHD = no structural disease; VT = ventricular tachycardia; WPW = Wolff-Parkinson-White (Modified with permission from Am J Cardiol 63:181, 1989.)

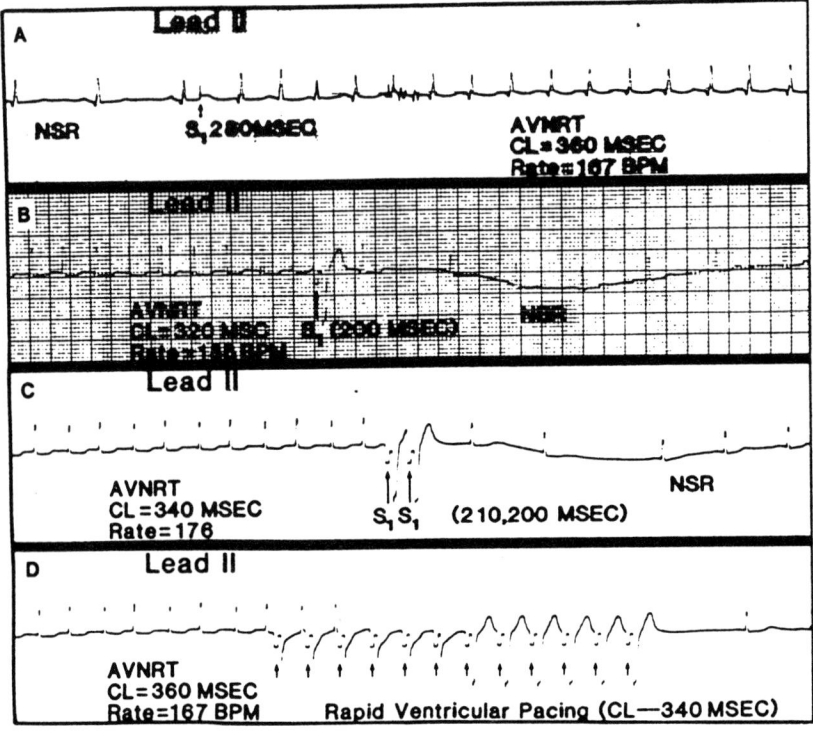

Figure 1: Patient 1. In panels A-D, lead II is shown with discontinuous rhythm strips. Panel A: normal sinus rhythm (NSR) is shown initially. A single endocardial extrastimulus (S_1) is delivered 280 msec after a sensed P wave through a permanent atrial lead used with an antitachycardia pacemaker. The extrastimulus induces atrioventricular nodal reentrant (AVNRT) with a cycle length of 360 msec or heart rate 167 ppm. Panel B: AVNRT with a rate of 188 ppm is terminated with a single external stimulus(S_1) coupled 200 msec after the QRS. Panel C: another episode of AVNRT with a rate of 176 ppm is terminated by double extrastimuli (S_1S_2) coupled in 210,200 msec after the QRS. Panel D: rapid ventricular pacing at a cycle length of 340 msec terminates a tachycardia with a rate of 167 ppm. (Reproduced with permission from Am J Cardiol, 63:180, 1989).

patient with atrioventricular nodal reentrant tachycardia all three attempts of external pacing resulted in arrhythmia termination with retrograde conduction of the premature ventricular impulse into the atrioventricular node. Atrial capture with transcutaneous pacing could not be documented in either of the two patients with atrioventricular nodal reentry or any of the nine with reciprocating tachycardia in whom external cardiac programmed stimulation was performed with an atrial electrode-catheter in place for endocardial recording.

A total of 187 episodes of orthodromic and 2 episodes of antidromic reciprocating SVT were studied in 10 patients with Wolff-Parkinson-White syndrome. In 9 of 10 patients, the tachycardia was terminated by external cardiac programmed stimulation. In 8 of these 9 patients, the SVT was reproducibly terminated between 2 and 100 times. In one patient, the protocol was discontinued because of intolerable discomfort that was reported by the patient after external pacing had successfully terminated a reciprocating tachycardia four times (patient 13). In the one patient (patient 4) in whom the technique was not successful, probably because of intermittent ventricular capture, the termination protocol was attempted six times. Overall, noninvasive transcutaneous cardiac programmed stimulation was successful in 179 of 189 (95%) episodes of reciprocating tachycardia and in 9 of 10 patients or in 198 of all 209 (95%) SVT episodes and in 11 of 13 patients.

Examples of tachycardia terminations of reciprocating tachycardia are shown in Figure 2. During this SVT with cycle length of 350 msec, a single extrastimulus with 210 msec coupling interval terminated the tachycardia in panel A. Atrial preexcitation is present with a premature atrial electrogram at 290 msec with subsequent antegrade block in the atrioventricular node. In panel B, double extrastimuli coupled in at 210 and 190 msec terminate the tachycardia.

Ventricular Tachycardia

Noninvasive transcutaneous cardiac programmed stimulation was attempted in 14 episodes of evoked VT in 9 patients. The technique was successful in terminating 5 of these 14 episodes. Eight patients had 9 episodes of VT with a cycle length <400 msec (rate >150 ppm). Two of these were successfully terminated with transcutaneous pacing. Four patients had a total of five tachycardias with cycle length >400 msec (rate <150 ppm). Three of these five tachycardias were terminated by transcutaneous pacing. Acceleration of one tachycardia occurred during external overdrive pacing and was terminated with endocardial pacing. Cardioversion or defibrillation was not required in any patient.

Figure 3 (panels A, B, and C) shows examples of VT terminations in separate patients. A single extrastimulus terminates a sustained

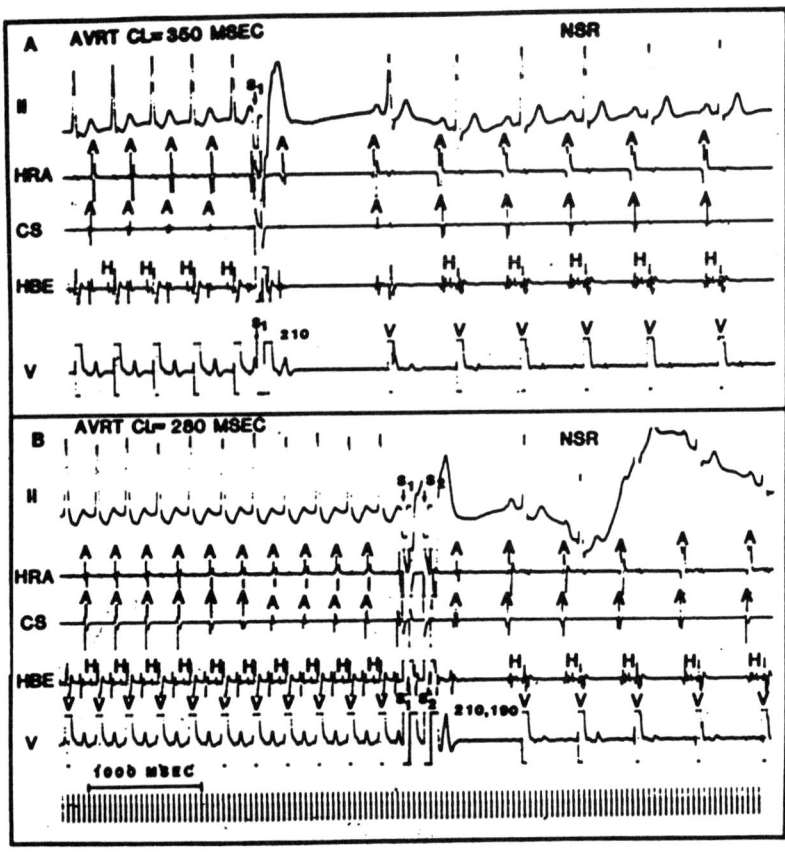

Figure 2. *Patient 5. Panel A: atrioventricular reciprocating tachycardia (AVRT) with cycle length 350 msec is shown with recordings from surface lead II and intracardiac recordings from the high right atrium (HRA), coronary sinus (CS), bundle of His (HBE) and ventricle (V). During the tachycardia, a single extrastimulus delivered 210 msec after a QRS results in capture of the ventricle. Retrograde conduction via the bypass tract to the atrium occurs with antegrade block in the atrioventricular node terminating the tachycardia with resumption of normal sinus rhythm (NSR). Panel B: the AVRT has accelerated to a cycle length of 280 msec after intravenous isoproterenol infusion. Double extrastimuli (S_1S_2), 210, and 190 msec after the QRS result in termination of the tachycardia. (Reproduced with permission from Am J Cardiol 63:180, 1989.)*

Sustained Supraventricular and Ventricular Tachycardias 141

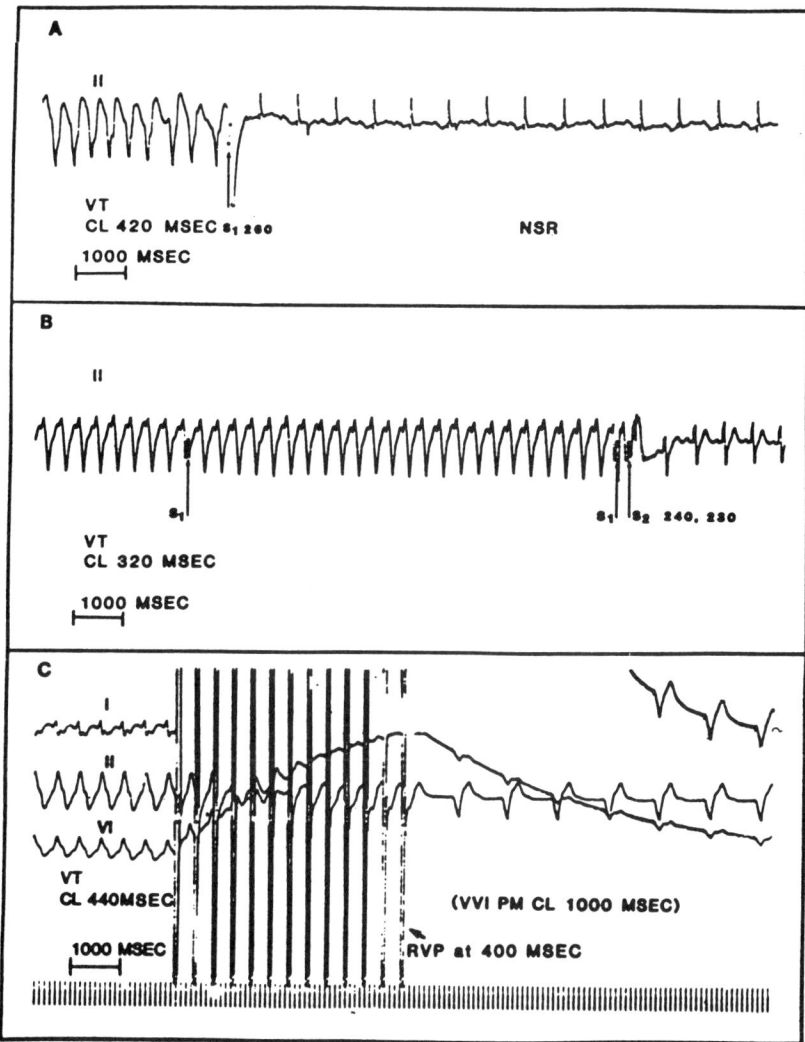

Figure 3: Panels A-C show three episodes of ventricular tachycardia (VT). Panel A: surface lead II is shown during a VT (420 msec) in patient 14. A single extrastimulus (S_1) coupled in 260 msec after a QRS terminates the tachycardia. Panel B: The initial extrastimulus (S_1) fails to capture the ventricle during an episode of VT with cycle length 320 msec in patient 16. Double extrastimuli (S_1S_2) coupled at 240, 230 msec results in tachycardia termination. Panel C: surface leads I, II, and V1 are shown during a tachycardia with cycle length of 440 msec in patient 15. Rapid ventricular pacing (RVP) at a cycle length of 400 msec terminates the tachycardia resulting in demand ventricular pacing (VVI PM) with a cycle length of 1000 msec. (Reproduced with permission from Am J Cardiol 63:181, 1989).

ventricular tachycardia in panel A. In panel B, a single extrastimulus (220 msec) fails to capture the ventricle, while two extrastimuli result in effective capture and termination of the tachycardia. In panel C, transcutaneous overdrive pacing successfully terminates the tachycardia. Distortion of surface leads I and V_1 is also noted in panel C contrasting with lead II where the modified preamplifiers in the noninvasive transcutaneous temporary pacemaker monitor eliminate the distortion.

Mode of Tachycardia Termination

With noninvasive transcutaneous cardiac programmed stimulation, of 20 episodes of atrioventricular nodal reentrant SVT, 12 were terminated with a single extrastimulus, 6 with double extrastimuli, 1 with overdrive rapid pacing, and 1 episode could not be terminated with transcutaneous pacing. Of 189 episodes of orthodromic reciprocating SVT, 156 were terminated with single extrastimuli, 22 with double extrastimuli, and one with overdrive pacing. External cardiac programmed stimulation was unsuccessful in 10 episodes of reciprocating SVT. Of 14 episodes of VT, one was terminated with a single extrastimulus, one with double extrastimuli, 3 with rapid pacing, and 9 could not be terminated.

Patient Discomfort

Of the 22 patients undergoing transcutaneous pacing, 19 had the procedure attempted on 1 occasion, 1 at 2 separate electrophysiological studies, and 2 at 3 studies. Thus there were a total of 27 ratings of discomfort by 22 patients. There were 4 reports of mild discomfort, 10 of moderate, 11 of severe, and 2 of intolerable discomfort that prompted discontinuation of the protocol. The patient discomfort reported had no relationship to stimulation threshold.

The mean threshold for ventricular capture with transcutaneous pacing was 68 ± 15 mA. In 21 of 27 times that transcutaneous pacing was performed in the 22 patients reliable ventricular capture was achieved during the tachycardia by stimulation at 5 mA over threshold. In 3 patients, it was necessary to increase the current by 10 mA, in 2 patients by 20 mA, and in one patient by 30 mA over threshold to achieve capture during the tachycardia.

Transcutaneous cardiac programmed stimulation was unsuccessful in terminating a sustained hemodynamically stable SVT on ten occasions and endocardial ventricular pacing had to be used for arrhythmia termination. On one occasion cardioversion was required when transcutaneous pacing and intravenous procainamide failed to terminate orthodromic reciprocating tachycardia in a patient with Wolff-Parkinson-White syndrome. When the transcutaneous technique failed, endocardial right ventricular pacing was used for VT termination in eight of nine episodes with one episode spontaneously terminating.

Discussion

Invasive Cardiac Programmed Stimulation for Arrhythmia Termination

Refinement of tachycardia termination techniques in the electrophysiology laboratory has led to the ability to interrupt most reentrant arrhythmias with endocardial pacing techniques.[1-5,16] Multiple factors such as mechanism and rate of the tachycardia, distance of the stimulation site from the reentrant circuit, conduction velocity and refractoriness of the intervening myocardium, and characteristics of the stimulus itself have been studied which determine whether pacing techniques will successfully interrupt the tachycardia during the termination zone.[3,14] Less clearly defined are the factors that contribute to arrhythmia acceleration. Nonetheless, the experience has been that single capture stimulation from an endocardial site results in arrhythmia acceleration in less than 1% of episodes, while multiple capture techniques or overdrive pacing cause acceleration in approximately 5% of termination attempts. However, single extrastimuli are not as effective in interrupting most tachycardias as multiple capture techniques.[4]

Noninvasive Transcutaneous Antitachycardic Pacing

Earlier attempts at noninvasive termination of SVT and VT with transcutaneous pacing were unsuccessful.[7] However, soon after these initial reports, termination of sustained monomorphic VT was achieved with use of external burst pacing at 180 ppm at maximal amplitude output (120 mA) with only minimal patient discomfort.[9] More recently, termination of sustained atrioventricular nodal reentrant tachycardia and VT was reported with use of burst pacing techniques.[12]

Noninvasive Transcutaneous Cardiac Programmed Stimulation

The standard external transcutaneous pacemaker required modifications to allow programmed stimulation with single or multiple extrastimuli and overdrive pacing with rates greater than 180 ppm. After initial feasibility studies of external cardiac programmed stimulation, we expanded our observations with particular emphasis on reciprocating tachycardias.[13] Because of the ease of induction and hemodynamic stability, this type of tachycardia is particularly suited to termination with external cardiac programmed stimulation.

Based on the experience with endocardial pacing, we designed a tiered protocol with transcutaneous cardiac programmed stimulation to terminate the tachycardias with the minimally effective stimulation.[16] This approach was also developed to minimize the risk of arrhythmia acceleration and reduce patient discomfort due to anxiety, and pectoralis muscle and cutaneous nerve stimulation. In our experience, patient tolerance of transcutaneous pacing is better with intermittent extrastimuli than with burst pacing.

Although not evaluated with this study, this modified device could be used for arrhythmia termination techniques such as underdrive pacing or delivering a drive train followed by extrastimuli. The potential applications of external cardiac programmed stimulation for noninvasive arrhythmia induction and assessment of drug efficacy are evident and merit further investigation.

Acknowledgment: The skilled assistance of Keith Mack, RN, Amy Payne, RN, and Gail Hamilton, are acknowledged with appreciation.

References

1. Wellens HJJ: Value and limitations of programmed electrical stimulation of the heart in the study and treatment of tachycardias. Circulation 57:845, 1978.

2. Ruddy R, Friday KJ, Southworth WF: Termination of ventricular tachycardia by single extrastimulation during the ventricular effective refractory period. Circulation 67:457, 1983.
3. Josephson ME, Horowitz LN, Farshidi A, et al.: Recurrent sustained ventricular tachycardia I. Mechanisms. Circulation, 57:431, 1978.
4. Fischer JD, Kim SG, Matos J, et al.: Comparative effectiveness of pacing techniques of well tolerated sustained ventricular tachycardia. PACE 6:915, 1983.
5. Waldo AL, McLen WAH: Treatment of cardiac arrhythmias with emphasis on cardiac pacing. *In:* Diagnosis and Treatment of Cardiac Arrhythmias Following Open Heart Surgery. Waldo, AL (ed). Futura Publishing Co., Mt Kisco, NY, 1980, p. 115.
6. Zoll PM: Resuscitation of the heart in ventricular standstill by external electrical stimulation. N Engl J Med 247:768, 1952.
7. Zoll PM, Zoll RH, Falk RH, et al.: External noninvasive temporary cardiac pacing: Clinical trials. Circulation 71:937, 1985.
8. Falk RH, Zoll PM, Zoll RH: Safety and efficacy of noninvasive cardiac pacing: A preliminary report. N Engl J Med 309:1166, 1983.
9. Rosenthal M, Stamato N, Marchlinsky F, et al.: Noninvasive cardiac pacing for termination of sustained, uniform ventricular tachycardia. Am J Cardiol 58:561, 1986.
10. Barold SS, Falkoff MD, Ong LS, et al.: Termination of ventricular tachycardia by transcutaneous cardiac pacing. Am Heart J 114:180, 1987.
11. Luck JC, Grubb BP, Artman SE, et al.: Termination of sustained ventricular tachycardia by external noninvasive pacing. Am J Cardiol 61:574, 1988.
12. Luck JC, Davis D: Termination of sustained tachycardia by external noninvasive pacing. PACE 10:1125, 1987.
13. Estes NAM III, Deering TF, Han EH, et al.: Noninvasive termination of sustained supraventricular and ventricular tachycardia with external cardiac programmed stimulation (abstr). J Am Coll Cardiol 9:200, 1987.
14. Waxman HL, Cain ML, Greenspan AM, et al.: Termination of ventricular tachycardia with ventricular stimulation: salutary effects of increased current strength. Circulation 65:800, 1982.
15. Estes NAM III, Deering TF, Manolis AS, et al.: External cardiac programmed stimulation for noninvasive termination of sustained supraventricular and ventricular tachycardia. Am J Cardiol 63:177, 1989.
16. Cameron J, Isner J, Salem D, et al.: Cardiac electrophysiologic testing: Its role in the supraventricular and ventricular arrhythmias. Pharmacotherapy 5:95, 1985.

VII

Echocardiographic Aspect

Chapter 13

Echocardiographic Evaluation of Left Ventricular Function During Noninvasive Transcutaneous Cardiac Pacing

Jan Kyst Madsen, MD, DMSc

Clinical studies have shown that noninvasive transcutaneous cardiac pacing (NTP or NTCP) is an effective procedure to restore heart rhythm in emergency situations.[1,2] In such acute situations, it is satisfactory to restore any pump function at all. However, the indications for noninvasive transcutaneous pacing is growing, and NTP has been used as stand-by during surgical procedures,[3] for overdrive pacing in patients with tachyarrhythmias,[4] and as substitution for a transvenous pacemaker for up to 14 hours.[2] In these circumstances, it is important that the myocardial pump function is retained or at least diminished only insignificantly during pacing.

The hemodynamic effect of NTP has been evaluated noninvasively with echocardiography and Doppler methods in healthy persons in two different studies.

Echocardiography

We evaluated ventricular function on 2D and M-mode echocardiography in ten volunteers.[5]

From *Noninvasive Transcutaneous Cardiac Pacing* edited by Pierre Birkui, M.D., Jacques Trigano, M.D., and Paul Zoll, M.D., © 1993, Futura Publishing Company, Inc., Mount Kisco, NY.

Material and Methods

Ten healthy volunteers, five men and five women, participated. They ranged in age from 23 to 33 years. Pacing with NTP was performed with a battery operated pacemaker, model 2011 (manufactured by S&W Medico Teknik A/S, Denmark). The pulse duration was 40 msec. Before the electrodes were positioned, the skin was carefully cleaned with alcohol, thereby removing salt and dust solved in the skin, which decreased the leaking current. The back electrode has 115 cm^2 in area. After the positive back electrode was put in place, the optimal position of the negative front electrode was determined, by moving the electrode until the position with the lowest threshold of stimulation was reached. After that the electrode was fixed to the skin. The front electrode has 75 cm^2 in area. All persons were paced for 30 mn, from 7.30 AM to 8.00 AM. The front electrode was placed just left on the lower part of the sternum and the back electrode to the left of the spine and below the left scapula. The pacemaker rate was set 10%-20% above resting heart rate, the output was then gradually increased until 100% capture was achieved, which was continued for 30 mn.

Echocardiography was performed with a General Electrique RT 3000 echocardiograph with combined motion-mode (M-mode) facility and phased array sector scanner (3.5 MHz) for two-dimensional (2D) presentation. M-mode and 2D presentations were stored on videotape for later analysis. All persons were studied in the left lateral decubitus position both during sinus rhythm and NTP. The M-mode presentation was used for measurement of left ventricular diameter at end-diastole (EED) and end-systole (ESD).[6] Left ventricular fractional shortening (FS) was calculated as follows: (EDD-ESD)/EDD × 100%. For 2D echocardiography, parasternal short and long axis views, and apical two-and four-chamber views were used. Left ventricular wall motion was judged by the overall visual impression after reviewing each study in real time, slow motion, and stop frame formats.

Results

The volunteers were paced with a rate from 85 to 115 ppm. The pace threshold for 100% pacing was from 38 to 70 mA. All were paced

Table 1.

	Sinus Rhythm		NTCP	
N	EDD (mm)	FS (%)	EDD (mm)	FS (%)
1	51	53	47	49
2	49	37	49	35
3	48	33	48	39
4	48	38	48	39
5	47	36	45	38
6	40	38	41	39
7	49	43	48	44
8	52	34	52	38
9	45	38	43	37
10	41	37	40	38
Mean (SD)	47 (4)	39 (6)	46 (4)	40 (4)
Normal range (6)	35–57	28–44		

Data from M-mode echocardiography during sinus rhythm and NTCP. EDD = left ventricular end-diastolic diameter; FS = fractional shortening. (Reproduced with permission from Madsen JK et al.[5])

without pain, though two felt slight chest discomfort and another two frequently coughed during pacing. Table 1 shows individual values of EED and fractional shortening. There were no significant changes in these parameters during pacing. Continuous M-mode examinations of the ventricle at the standard projection during sinus rhythm and NTCP revealed no major differences between the contraction patterns of the interventricular septum and the posterior wall. This was the same whether sinus rhythm preceded paced rhythm or vice versa. There was synchronous contraction and no paradoxical movement or early systolic anterior or posterior movement of the interventricular septum during NTCP (Figs. 1, 2).

This contraction pattern is in contrast to the findings during endocardial pacing, where an echocardiographic pattern similar to bundle branch block is found. This indicates a simultaneous contraction of the ventricles during NTP.

Figure 3 shows that the normal anterior movement, the A wave, of the mitral valve during diastole (i.e., atrial systole) disappears during NTCP. This indicates that the atrium is stimulated either simultaneous with the ventricles or retrograde.

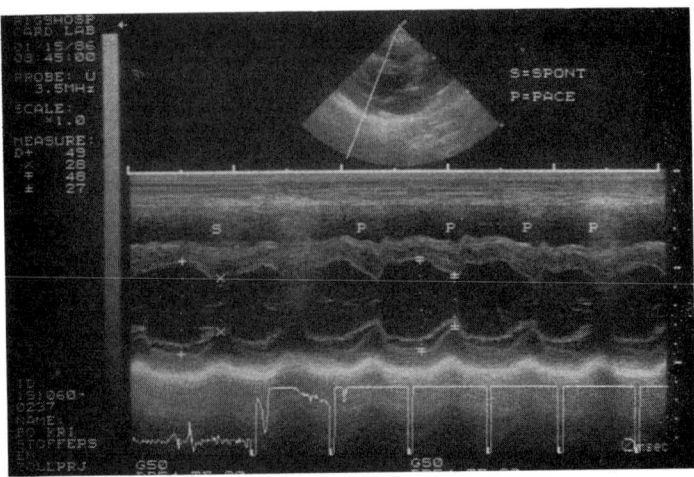

Figure 1. M-mode echocardiogram at the standard projection demonstrating normal left ventricular contraction pattern during transition from sinus rhythm (S) to transcutaneous pacing (P). (Reproduced with permission from Madsen JK, et al.[5])

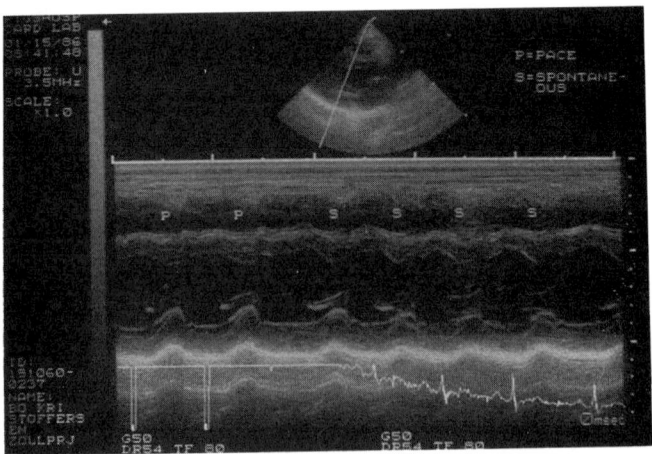

Figure 2. M-mode echocardiogram at the standard projection demonstrating normal left ventricular contraction pattern during transition from transcutaneous pacing (P) to sinus rhythm (S). (Reproduced with permission from Madsen JK, et al.[5])

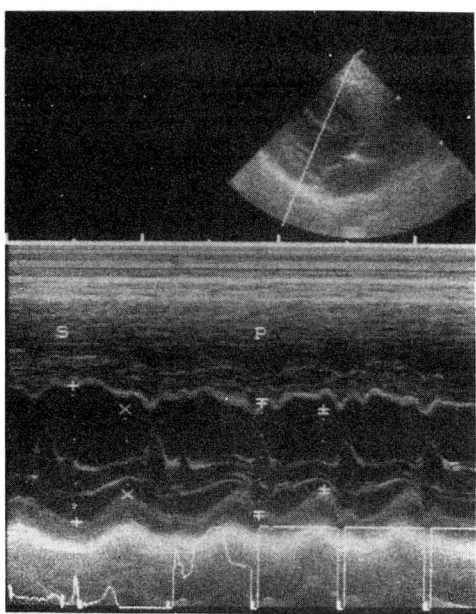

Figure 3. M-mode echocardiogram of the mitral valve during transition from sinus rhythm (S) to transcutaneous pacing (P). Note the disappearance of the A waves during pacing, indicating the lack of an atrial systole. (Reproduced with permission from Madsen JK, et al.[5])

Doppler Assessment

Talit et al. performed continuous-wave Doppler evaluation on ten normal subjects during sinus rhythm and under NTP[7] (Fig. 4).

Material and Methods

The volunteers were paced with a Zoll NTP (ZMI Corporation, Woburn, MA, USA). The pacing was performed through a negative anterior electrode on the lower left sternal area, and a positive posterior electrode on the left subscapular area.

Doppler measurements were obtained from the suprasternal notch with a 2.5 MHz continuous wave transducer. After the optimal position was obtained during sinus rhythm, the transducer was kept in this position for the rest of the study. Only the highest velocities obtained were used.

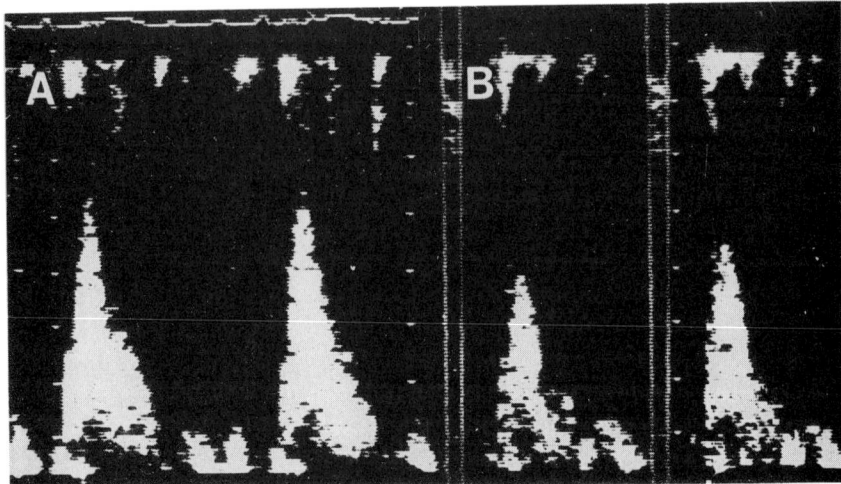

Figure 4. *Continuous wave Doppler of the aortic outflow during sinus rhythm (A) and during transcutaneous pacing (B) in the same individual. Note the smaller peak velocity and flow integral during pacing. (Reproduced with permission from Talit U et al.[7])*

The index of stroke volume (ISV) was taken as the integral of the area under the aortic flow velocity curve obtained from the Doppler tracing. The index of cardiac output (ICO) as shown in Figure 4 was calculated as the product of the ISV and the heart rate.

Doppler measurements were initially obtained during sinus rhythm. The output of the NTP was gradually increased until a stable pacing rhythm, only slightly above the subjects intrinsic rate was reached.

Results

The subjects were paced, on average, 13% above their own resting sinus rhythm.

Capture was obtained by NTCP with a mean threshold of 61 ± 15 mA. Nine out of the ten subjects tolerated pacing easily. In the last subject, pacing was terminated immediately after data collection due to the chest discomfort at a threshold of 100 mA.

Table 2 shows the individual values of heart rate, index of stroke

Table 2.

N	Heart Rate (ppm) SR	NTCP	Stroke Volume (ml/m2) SR	NTCP	Cardiac Output (ml/m2) SR	NTCP	%
1	84	101	16.6	14.4	1394	1454	+4
2	90	101	16.7	14.6	1503	1474	−2
3	80	76	15.8	12.1	1264	919	−28
4	82	78	22.9	16.0	1877	1248	−34
5	65	83	20.2	15.6	1313	1294	−2
6	65	86	20.7	12.4	1345	1066	−21
7	68	75	21.0	17.9	1428	1342	−6
8	69	74	19.1	16.7	1317	1237	−6
9	61	77	16.0	9.6	976	739	−24
10	66	69	8.5	6.4	561	442	−21
Mean	73	82	17.7	13.5	1297	1121	−14

Doppler estimated indices of stroke volume and cardiac output during sinus rhythm (SR) and cardiac pacing (NTCP) in 10 normal subjects. (Reproduced with permission from Talit U et al.[7])

volume, and index of cardiac output. The mean stroke volume was down by 24% during pacing, but due to the higher heart rate during pacing, the index of cardiac output was only decreased by 14% when compared to its value in sinus rhythm. In Figure 4, typical changes in Doppler flow during pacing are shown.

Discussion

It would be logical to assume an impaired function of the left ventricle during NTCP. One reason could be the altered sequence of stimulation of the atria and ventricles. As shown in Figure 3, the atrial systole is missing during NTP. This is in accordance with studies of the electrocardiogram by an esophageal electrode, during NTCP.[8] This showed that the pacing was ventricular in all cases and that the activation of the atria was retrograde. This sequence of activation is expected to cause a decrease in left ventricular pump function.

The echocardiographic study (Table 1) showed no impairment of the left ventricular function during NTCP. However, the stroke volume index was decreased by 23.5% during NTCP compared to its value in sinus rhythm, when measured by the Doppler method (Table 2). The heart rate during NTCP was higher than during sinus rhythm, which compensated for the decreased stroke volume, so the fall in cardiac index was only 14%. Though the fall was statistically significant, it is only a minor fall seen from a clinical viewpoint. This is further stressed by the unchanged echocardiographic findings and furthermore by an unchanged systolic and diastolic blood pressure during pacing.[5]

Both the cited studies[5,7] were performed on healthy volunteers. The situation may be different in patients. Feldman et al.[9] performed NTCP during catheterization on 16 patients with angina. The patients were paced at a heart rate of 85% of the predicted maximum rate. During maximal pacing all patients showed a rise in atrial, pulmonary artery, and mean aortic pressures. However, such a pace rate is usually never used.

Conclusion

The function of the left ventricle is only slightly impaired during NTP in healthy persons. Most likely the situation is the same in patients with heart disease though, for the time being, this has not been proved. However, even a modest decrease in pump function is of course of no importance in a life threatening situation. In more selective cases, such as described in the introduction, it is the impression that the left ventricular function is sufficiently preserved so that NTCP may be used without further considerations on pump function.

References

1. Zoll PM, Zoll RH, Falk RH, et al.: External noninvasive temporary cardiac pacing: Clinical trials. Circulation 71:937, 1985.
2. Madsen JK, Meibom J, Videbaek R, et al.: Transcutaneous pacing: Experience with the Zoll noninvasive temporary pacemaker. Am Heart J 116:7, 1988.
3. Berliner D, Okun M, Peters RW, et al.: Transcutaneous temporary pacing in operating room. JAMA 254:84, 1985.
4. Luck JC, Grubb BP, Artman SE, et al.: Termination of sustained ventricular tachycardia by external noninvasive pacing. Am J Cardiol 61:574, 1988.
5. Madsen K, Pedersen F, Grande P, et al.: Normal myocardial enzymes and normal echocardiographic findings during noninvasive transcutaneous pacing. PACE 11:1188, 1988.

6. Feigenbaum H: Echocardiography, 4th edition. Lea & Febiger, Philadelphia, 1986.
7. Talit U, Leach CN, Werner MS, et al.: The effect of external cardiac pacing on stroke volume. PACE 13:598, 1990.
8. Falk RH, Ngai STA, Kumaki DJ, et al.: Cardiac activation during external cardiac pacing. PACE 10:503, 1987.
9. Feldman MD, Zoll PM, Aroeasty JM, et al.: Hemodynamic response to noninvasive external cardiac pacing. Am J Med 84:395, 1988.

VIII

New Applications

Chapter 14

New Clinical Applications of Noninvasive Transcutaneous Cardiac Pacing

Fryderyk Prochaczek, MD, Jerzy Galecka,
Krzysztof Jarczok, MD

A modified method of noninvasive transcutaneous cardiac pacing (NTCP), introduced into clinical practice in 1981, was used for effective ventricular pacing in conscious subjects without the need for analgesic drugs.[1-4] The modified method resulted in the ability to check the electrical response of ventricles to stimulating impulses. The advantages of modified transcutaneous heart stimulation can be widely applied in clinical practice. The first trials of transcutaneous cardiac pacing for choosing antiarrhythmic drugs for fast atrial and ventricular dysrhythmias and for diagnostic purposes have been completed.[4-8] The aim of this study was the evaluation of the usefulness of transcutaneous heart stimulation for the following: (1) noninvasive testing of ventriculo-atrial conduction; (2) protection and diagnostics of carotid sinus hypersensitivity of the cardioinhibitory type; (3) estimation of coronary reserve.

Transcutaneous Heart Pacing: Testing Ventriculo-atrial Conduction

In 1987, Falk et al.[9] and Klein et al.[10] showed that transcutaneous heart stimulation in men excites only the ventricles, and excitation of

From *Noninvasive Transcutaneous Cardiac Pacing* edited by Pierre Birkui, M.D., Jacques Trigano, M.D., and Paul Zoll, M.D., © 1993, Futura Publishing Company, Inc., Mount Kisco, NY.

the atria occurs via retrograde conduction through the atrio-ventricular node. It enables a noninvasive estimation of ventriculo-atrial conduction as long as registration of atrial excitation from the esophagus during the course of transcutaneous heart stimulation is carried out.

Materials and Methods

Fifteen healthy volunteers, aged 20 to 58 (mean age: 40 years), were tested after obtaining their consent. All tests were carried out with equipment for cardioversion and drug therapy reanimation ready for use. For the electrophysiologic tests, a noninvasive transcutaneous NP-4D (Demand) cardiostimulator (Obream-Temed, Poland) and high impedance electrodes (each surface area 50 cm^2, made by Obream-Temed) were used (Fig. 1). With the cardiostimulator, it

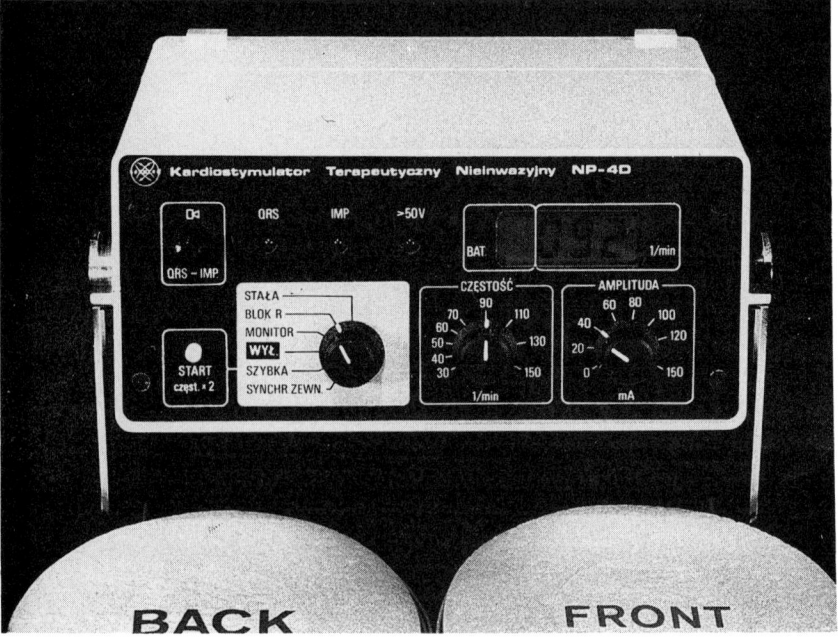

Figure 1. *A noninvasive transcutaneous external stimulator (NP-4D, Obream-Temed, Poland). The stimulator provides legible recordings, compatible with every type of cardiomonitor and ECG recorder.*

was possible to pace with a frequency up to 250 ppm and a rectangular stimulating impulse lasting 30 msec with a current intensity up to 150 mA. The NP-4D stimulator comprises an elimination system of the artefact of the stimulating impulse, and for experimental purposes, it can be switched "on" and "off." Impulse of the stimulator and duration of the suppression are shown on the ECG recording as an oscillation of 100-Hz frequency and deviation of about 2 mm. Figure 2 shows dependance of the regulated suppression time on the shape of the paced QRS.[11] The above described system enables legible recordings from any bipolar ECG lead to be received. This facilitates the use of transcutaneous heart stimulation for diagnostic purposes.

Before beginning transcutaneous ventricular pacing, a bipolar "capsule" electrode (distance between stimulating electrodes: 2 cm) was positioned in the esophagus after the gelatine capsule dissolved. The "capsule" electrode was swallowed while sipping water. The electrode was positioned to obtain the highest amplitude of left atrium excitation during the course of transcutaneous ventricular pacing.

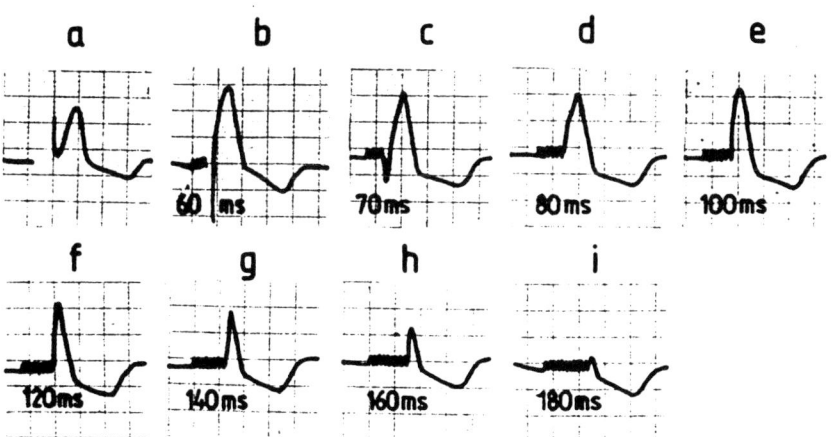

Figure 2. *Influence of the artefact suppression time of the stimulation impulse on the shape of paced QRS complex:* **a.** *Recording of stimulation without artefact suppression (switched "off")–writing hands went beyond recording range;* **b, c.** *Suppression time of 50 and 60 msec (the artefact diminished but writing hands continue to work incorrectly);* **d, e.** *Suppression time of 80 and 100 msec. Optimum shape of the recorded QRS complex accompanied with normal work of writing hands;* **f, g, h, i.** *Suppression time of 120, 140, 160, and 180 msec. Influence on the shape of the recorded QRS complex (Pacer speed 50 mm/sec).*

To prove the efficacy of transcutaneous heart pacing, a sphygmogram from the right common carotid artery was recorded. Before stimulation, a negative stimulating electrode was placed on the anterior chest surface in place of the V_3 (for ECG) and the positive was placed between the spinal column and scapula corresponding to V_3. During examination, ventricular excitation and toleration thresholds were estimated. Heart rhythm control from the cardiostimulator was established when the carotid sphygmogram waves were consistent with electrode impulses. The ventricle excitation threshold was taken to be the lowest value of the stimulating impulse current that achieved 100% frequency agreement between stimulating impulses and sphygmoram waves. The tolerance threshold was taken to be the highest current stimulating impulse amplitude that the patient could sustain.

In the diagnostic procedures, i.e., tests of ventriculo-atrial conduction, ventricles were paced with a current intensity 20% higher than the ventricle excitation threshold. In all tested subjects, the posterior-anterior measurement of the chest was taken at the level of the xiphoid process (supine position).

Results

Effective ventricular stimulation was achieved in 10 of 15 (67%) volunteers. The postero-anterior measurement of subjects that had effective ventricular stimulation was, on average, 23 cm as compared to 21.5 cm for the whole group. The average ventricular excitation threshold equaled 42 mA (range : 22 to 72 mA) and was much lower than the average toleration threshold of 70 mA (range : 50 to 90 mA). In 8 of the 10 subjects with effective transcutaneous ventricular stimulation, retrograde atria activation was found (Figs. 3–5). In the remaining two subjects, atria activations of sinus origin were found. A retrograde II degree atrioventricular block of Mobitz type I was seen at a mean heart rate of 156 ppm on average.

Discussion

Transcutaneous heart stimulation of conscious subjects without the use of analgesic drugs is limited by the tolerance threshold of the patient. The examination itself has been well tolerated as the ventricle excitation threshold (average 42 mA) was much lower than the

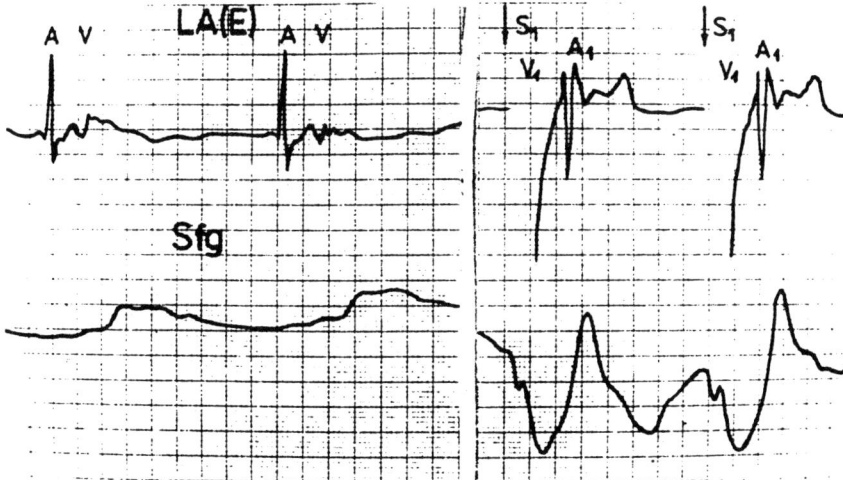

Figure 3. A comparison between the ECG and the sphygmogram (Sfg) obtained during sinus rhythm and during effective NTCP (S_1). **A, V**: recordings of atria and ventricle excitation of sinus origin; S_1: stimulator impulse; V_1, A_1: recordings of ventricle and retrograde atrial excitation; **LA/E**: esophageal ECG taken from the left atrium level. Suppression system "off."

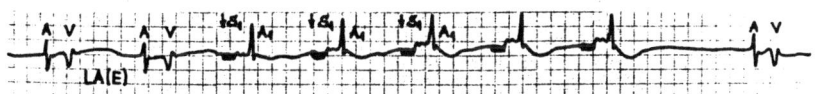

Figure 4. ECG recording from esophageal lead at the level of the left atrium (LA/E) when the unit for suppression of the artefact of the stimulating impulse is switched "on." S_1: stimulation impulse marker; A_1: retrograde atrial activation with a slight ventricular activation.

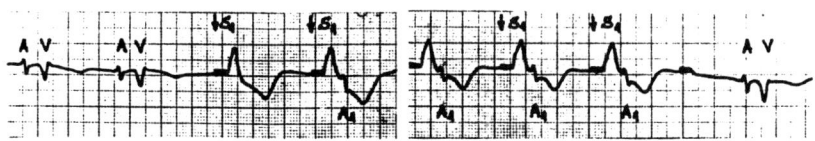

Figure 5. Switching "on" and "off" of the NTCP registered in bipolar esophago-thoracal lead. Both the retrograde atrial activation (A_1-A_1) and the distinct ventricular activation are registered.

mean toleration threshold of the transcutaneous ventricular stimulation (70 mA).

The quality of the recordings during transcutaneous ventricular stimulation from the bipolar esophageal lead distinguished between atria stimulation of sinus origin and atria stimulation from the ventricle side. The results confirmed that at the stimulating impulse currents used in this work, ventricles are stimulated first and then the atria by retrograde excitation passing through the AV junction.

As shown schematically in Figure 6, the ventricles are closer to the active electrode (V_3) than the atria. The ventricles are in the highest electric potential field that is sufficient to start ventricular excitation. Atria lie outside of this field, and this study has shown that with stimulating pulses of 42 mA on average, the atria are not stimulated.

In this work with transcutaneous ventricle stimulation, it was possible to show a ventriculo-atrial conduction in 80% of the subjects

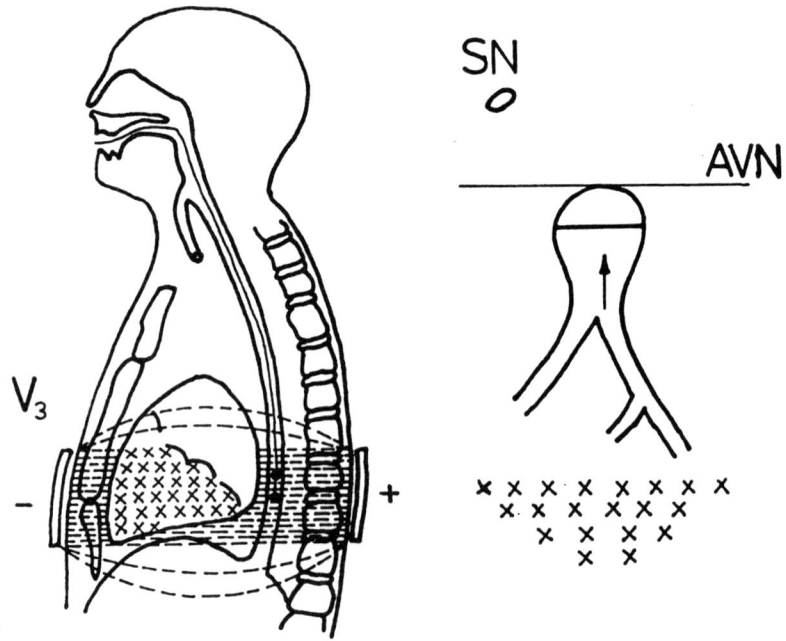

Figure 6. *The scheme of a transcutaneous and "capsule" electrode localization. Dotted lines = probable current density.* **X**: *ventricular activation;* **AVN**: *atrioventricular node.*

tested. This is consistent with the results of ventriculo-atrial conduction seen in healthy subjects tested using transesophageal ventricular stimulation.[12]

In addition, the efficiency of retrograde ventriculo-atrial conduction measured as the onset of the II ventriculoatrial block of Mobitz type I was similar to that seen in healthy subjects.[12] It should be emphasized that the effective transcutaneous ventricular stimulation that was achieved in the 10 tested subjects had larger antero-posterior chest measurements (23 cm on average) than the 15 subject group as a whole (21.5 cm).

This suggests the possibility of employing transcutaneous ventricular stimulation for assessing ventriculo-atrial conduction in subjects with large measurements in whom effective ventricular stimulation through the transesophageal route usually is impossible.[12]

The described possibility of recording atria activation in the course of transcutaneous ventricular stimulation suggests the use of the method for evaluating ventriculo-atrial conduction.

Transcutaneous Heart Stimulation for Diagnosis of Hypertensive Carotid Sinus Syndrome of The Cardioinhibitory Type

Using the carotid sinus stimulation test requires that immediate heart stimulation is available in case of prolonged asystole. This is especially necessary for carotid sinus hypersensitivity in which carotid sinus massage causes asystole due to sinus arrest and third degree AV block.[13-14]

Introduction by Stryjer et al.[14] of a new classification based on electrophysiologic heart investigation made the diagnosis of this syndrome more precise.

The aim of this part of the study was the verification of the diagnostic usefulness and safety of performing transcutaneous ventricular stimulation and transesophageal atrial stimulation for diagnosis of carotid sinus hypersensitivity of the cardioinhibitory type.

Materials and Methods

Twenty patients with syncope due to carotid sinus hypersensitivity classified for pharmacological treatment were included in this study. The mean age of the patients was 62 years. Among them were 18 men and 2 women. The patients were chosen after prior confirmation of the efficacy of transcutaneous ventricular stimulation. The average ventricular excitation threshold equaled 60 mA (from 44 to 75 mA).

Estimation of the cardioinhibitory type of the carotid sinus hypersensitivity was based on the electrophysiological studies introduced by Stryjer et al.[14] and adopted by us for noninvasive heart stimulation. Type A of the cardioinhibitory syndrome was characterized by sinus node inhibition during carotid sinus massage. Type B was characterized by complete AV block, and type C was characterized by combined sinus node inhibition and complete AV block.

Atrial or ventricular stimulation was started in the third second of asystole caused by sinus massage. Atria were stimulated with the use of an SP-5 transesophageal stimulator, and ventricles were stimulated with a transcutaneous NP-4D stimulator (Obream-Temed, Poland). In the event of sinus arrest, sinus carotid massage was repeated during transesophageal atrial stimulation and during transcutaneous ventricle stimulation. In the course of examination, bipolar esophageal leads were recorded from the level of the left atrium and bipolar leads from the surface of the chest from RV_6 and V_6 points. Because this lead is perpendicular to the route of the stimulating impulse current, a much more diminished artefact of the stimulating impulse is registered on the ECG. The lead from the chest was additionally protected against disturbances by the NP-4D stimulator in the manner described above.

Results

In 17 of 20 tested subjects, massage of the carotid sinus caused sinus arrest (Fig. 7). In 10 subjects, in the course of atrial stimulation, atrioventricular conduction was 1:1, a complete AV block occurred in 7 subjects. In all subjects of this group, effective heart stimulation by the transcutaneous route was achieved. The esophageal ECG recording showed no retrograde atrial activation (Fig. 8). In 3 of 20 tested subjects, carotid sinus massage caused only complete AV block and effective pacing by transcutaneous stimulation was achieved. No retrograde atrial activation was found in the esophageal ECG

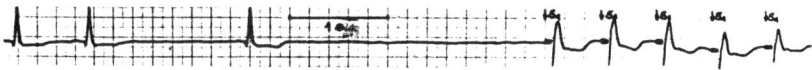

Figure 7. Sinus arrest caused by carotid sinus massage with effective NTCP and registered with a bipolar lead from the chest (paper speed 50 mm/sec).

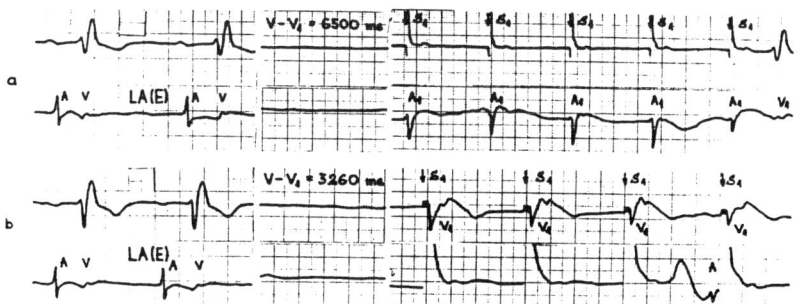

Figure 8. Heart asystole caused by carotid sinus massage followed by: **a.** Effective transesophageal atrial stimulation (S_1A_1) with blocked conduction to the ventricles. **b.** Transcutaneous ventricular stimulation (S_1V_1). In esophageal recording (LA/E), no electrical activity of atria in the first period.

recording. Figure 9 shows the obtained results and the diagnostic procedures.

Discussion

Introduced by Stryjer et al.,[14] diagnosis of the cardioinhibitory type of carotid sinus hypersensitivity requires heart cathetherization. Therefore, it is an invasive method. The method is accurate and protects the patient against uncontrolled asystole triggered by the doctor. In many cases the examination has to be repeated prior to pacemaker implantation. Therefore, it is reasonable to test for carotid sinus with noninvasive methods that are less expensive.

The obtained results indicate that in 50% (10 out of 20) of tested subjects displaying the cardioinhibitory type of carotid sinus hypersensitivity, it was necessary to stimulate the ventricles. A similar rate of ventricular stimulation during examination of carotid sinus hypersensitivity by invasive methods was shown by Stryjer (20 out of 38 patients). In our study, ventricular pacing was achieved in all

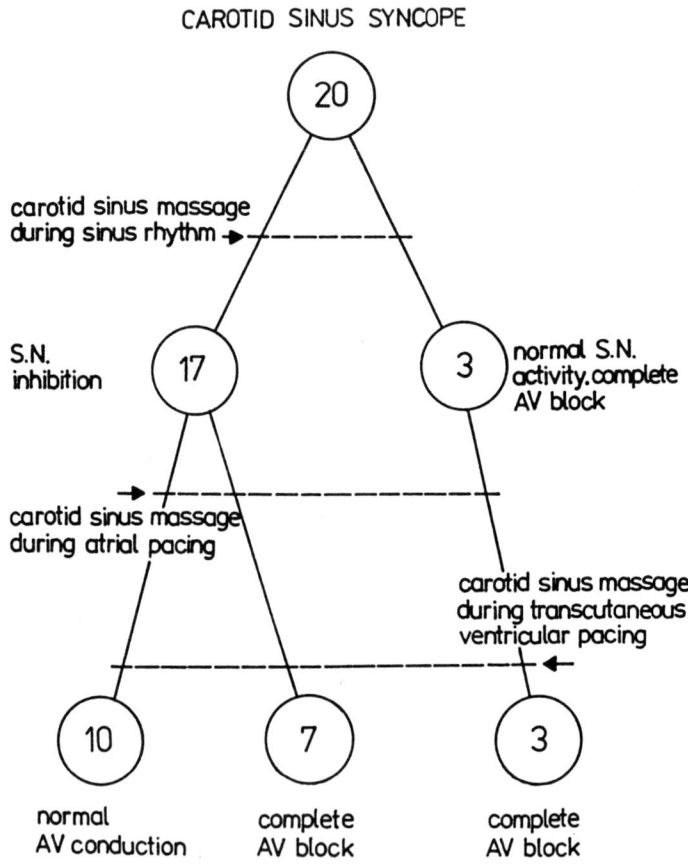

Figure 9. *A cardiodepressive response to carotid sinus massage during sinus rhythm and during transesophageal atrial stimulation and NTCP.*

subjects by transcutaneous heart stimulation. It should be noted that only patients in whom transcutaneous stimulation was effective were included. It seems that transcutaneous ventricular stimulation may effectively protect the patient against ventricular asystole.

Transesophageal atrial stimulation and transcutaneous heart stimulation differentiated particular types of cardioinhibitory response to carotid sinus stimulation with an accuracy similar to endocavitary heart stimulation. Similar to Stryjer's study, we found that types A and C carotid sinus hypersensitivity were most common. The accuracy of noninvasive methods revealed depressed retrograde conduction to the atria in types B and C. Summing up, we may assume that the electrophysiological examination of carotid sinus hypersensitivity of the cardioinhibitory type is both possible and safe with the noninvasive method.

Coronary Reserve Estimation Based on Transcutaneous Heart Stimulation : Comparison with Exercise and Stimulation Tests

Noninvasive diagnosis of coronary insufficiency in subjects who don't reveal ECG features of ischemia is based on tests increasing oxygen demand by the heart. It can be achieved by increasing muscle work (effort test) or by increasing heart work (electrical stimulation). Increase of heart work only can be achieved by increasing heart rate with endocavitary or transesophageal stimulation (controlled tachycardia).

The aim of the study was to compare ECG features of heart ischemia at maximal heart rate obtained either with transesophageal or transcutaneous heart stimulation and with a classical exercise test.

Material and Methods

In 10 men with proved effort angina, retrosternal pain triggered by effort of NYHA II/III level, and a normal resting ECG, a coronary test was carried out on consecutive days using a cycloergometric test and transesophageal and transcutaneous stimulations. The average age of subjects was 58 years (range: 45 to 64).

In the first stage of testing, patients were loaded with increasing work until chest pain occurred. In coronary stimulatory tests, patients were stimulated for 3 min with a rate of 130 ppm. The stimulation was interrupted when a constant chest pain occurred that was different from knocking caused by transcutaneous heart stimulation and burning caused by transesophageal stimulation. The average atrial excitation threshold equaled 8 mA (range : 5 to 10 mA). For five patients, transesophageal stimulation was unnoticeable due to a lower atrial excitation threshold than noticeable stimulation. The average ventricular excitation threshold by NTCP equaled 55 mA (range : 38 to 65 mA). Atria and ventricles were stimulated with a current amplitude 20% higher than their excitation threshold. All tests were performed 72 hours after withdrawal from drugs that would affect the heart. During the exercise test, a 12-lead resting ECG was recorded immediately after the exercise and every 30 sec until normalization of the ECG recording. In transesophageal stimulation, a 12-lead ECG was recorded after every minute of stimulation and every 15 sec after its completion until pathological recording was normalized. ECG recording was not done during transcutaneous stimulation due to enormous disturbances caused by stimulating impulses. ECG recordings were registered immediately after completion of stimulation and every 15 sec until normalization of the ECG recording. Before switching "off" stimulation, an ECG recorder was switched "on" in order to receive a legible, undisturbed recording immediately after switching "off" stimulation. In every test, the moment of pain relief and normalization of ECG recording was registered.

Results

Exercise testing provoked retrosternal pain in every tested patient after work equal to an average of 3200 kg. Transesophageal stimulation induced retrosternal pain in one patient in the second minute and in other patients in the third minute of examination. NTCP caused retrosternal pain in two patients in the second minute and in eight other patients in the third minute of examination. In all examined patients, applied coronary tests caused mean ST segment depression of 0.3 mV (range: 0.2 to 0.5 mV). The most expressed and most frequent alterations could be found in leads V_2 to V_6 (Figs. 10, 11). Retrosternal pain caused by transesophageal stimulation retreated on average 10 sec after its completion, 30 sec after NTCP, and

New Clinical Applications 173

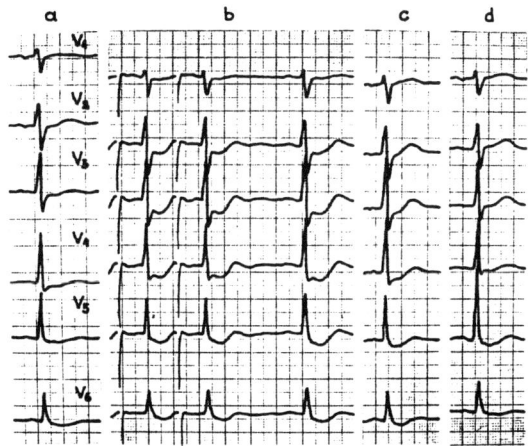

Figure 10. *Transesophageal positive coronary test:* **a.** *Resting ECG;* **b.** *At the moment of switching "on." Stimulation depression of ST segment by 0.5 mV in V_3, V_4;* **c, d.** *Recording 15 and 30 sec later after switching "off" stimulation.*

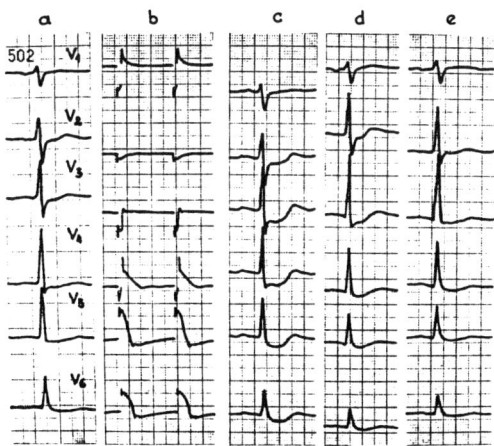

Figure 11. *Transcutaneous positive coronary test:* **a.** *resting ECG;* **b.** *recording during the course of stimulation with pressed ECG block;* **c.** *recording immediately after switching "off." Stimulation-depression of the ST segment of 0.5 mV in V_3, V_4;* **d, e.** *recording 30 and 45 sec later after switching "off" stimulation.*

174 NONINVASIVE TRANSCUTANEOUS CARDIAC PACING

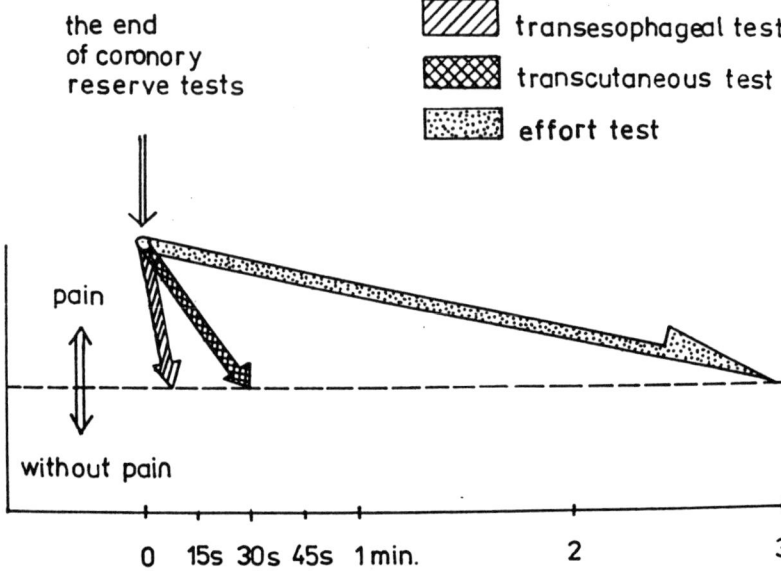

Figure 12. *The rate of pain disappearing in relation to the type of coronary test.*

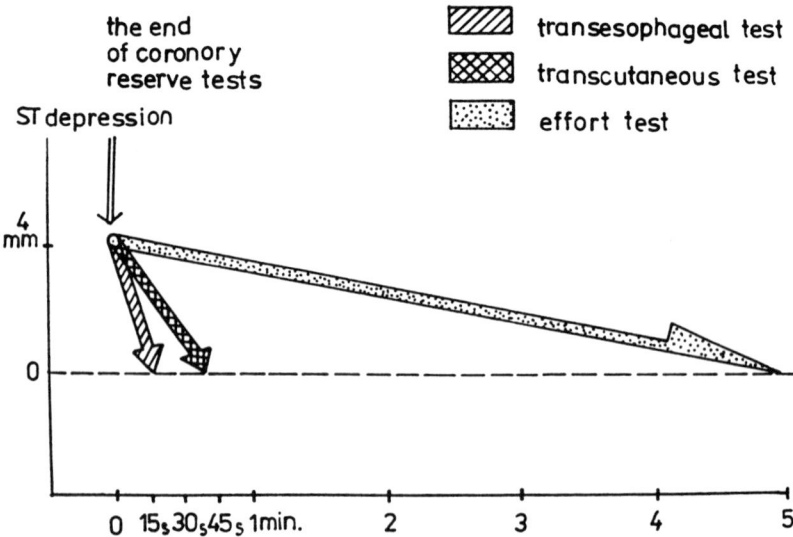

Figure 13. *The rate of normalization of ST segment placement in relation to the type of coronary test.*

3 min after exercise testing (Fig. 12). A similar tendency after completion of the tests could be observed in ST segment level depression. After transesophageal stimulation, a normalization of the ST segment level was observed on average after 15 sec, after NTCP after 40 sec on average, and after exercise testing only in the fifth minute on average (Fig. 13).

Discussion

Transcutaneous heart stimulation resulted in fast, usually strong knocking against the anterior chest wall and was tolerated for 3 min by all tested subjects. These complaints caused no major problems and preparing and performing the test was very simple. Therefore, the test shows superiority to the exercise test and transesophageal stimulation. A disadvantage of the test is that is is not possible to monitor ST segment level changes during stimulation due to aberrant conduction (ventricular excitation) or absence of a stimulator protecting 12 ECG leads against disturbances caused by a stimulating impulse. The stimulation test provoked retrosternal pain and similar ST segment depression in all examined patients. It provided a similar heart ischemia caused by the three compared coronary tests. The fact that a positive coronary test was obtained in all subjects after each of the tests performed is due to the fact that patients with restricted coronary reserve were chosen for the study. This was done to perform the coronary test as fast as possible and with the lowest frequency per minute. Interesting differences are noted between these tests as far as rate of disappearance of pain and depression of ST segment. The most rapid regression is observed after transesophageal stimulation because only the heart is forced to perform the more intensive work. Differences in the period of the appearing pain and ST segment deviations may not be the result only of unnoticeable ECG differences in degree of heart ischemia caused by coronary tests. In an exercise test, a higher heart rate and intensity of heart work are due to the work of large muscles of the lower limbs where an oxygen deficit may sometimes occur. The oxygen deficit and concomitant rise in blood presure forces a more intensive workload on the heart for a certain period after the test is completed. This may explain why in the exercise test, which causes a similar degree of ischemia as stimulation tests, ischemia disappears after a longer time period. In the transcutaneous test, unlike the transesophageal coronary test, skeletal muscles, mainly chest muscles, are stimulated too. To a certain degree, it may explain the slower rate of the disappearance of ischemia in the NTCP test compared to the transesophageal test. On the other hand, the reason for a slower disappearance of ischemia may result from a more intense ischemia caused by ventricular stimulation because retrosternal pain appears earlier during transcutaneous testing than during transesophageal coronary testing. A direct cause of the more intensive ischemia in the transcutaneous test also may be the impairment of the coronary flow during ventricular stimulation.[15]

The results of the transcutaneous coronary test are encouraging. It may be particularly useful in subjects with low ventricular excitation threshold in which exclusion or confirmation of restriction of coronary reserve is needed.

Conclusion

Based on the results of the new clinical application of NTCP, one may optimistically look into the future for their application in clinical cardiology.

A noninvasive estimation of ventriculo-atrial conduction may become very useful for the selection of the optimal mode of pacing in patients with no need of invasive electrophysiology to confirm the permanent pacing indication. Using various periods of time, on different days, and with various drugs, this method may substantially document several types of retroconduction.

Efficient and quick estimation of the hypersensitive carotid sinus, one of the important causes of transient brain and heart ischemia, has important implications for patient outcome. Examination via endocavitary stimulation reduces only a priori the number of subjects to be examined, restricted not only by the technology available in the electrophysiology laboratory but by the necessity of obtaining a patient's consent, complications, and the high cost of the examination. In comparison to invasive examination, the diagnostic test with NTCP may be performed safely and with similar accuracy in outpatient clinics for a large number of patients. Therefore, diagnostic testing with NTCP eliminates a substantial limitation of an invasive method of carotid sinus hypersensitivity diagnosis. It seems likely that this noninvasive test soon will be used in clinical practice for diagnosis and safe control of patients with hypersensitive carotid sinus syndrome.

The value of the NTCP test in coronary reserve estimation may at first arouse more doubts than new possibilities of clinical NTCP application. The coronary NTCP test was well tolerated and displayed a similar accuracy in revealing atherosclerotic ischemia as diagnostic tests used thus far. Taking into consideration that our last observations didn't reveal diminished examination sensivitity by shortening its duration down to 60 sec, one may assume that NTCP testing will become a valuable tool in clinical cardiology as a preliminary and quick method for selection of patients for invasive cardiology.

References

1. Zoll PM: Resuscitation of the heart in ventricular standstill by external electrical stimulation. N Engl J Med 247:768, 1952.
2. Zoll RH, Zoll PM, Belgard A: External noninvasive electrical stimulation of the heart. Crit Care Med 9:393, 1981.
3. Zoll PM, Zoll RH, Falk RH, et al.: External temporary cardiac pacing: Clinical trials. Circulation 71:937, 1985.
4. Zoll PM: Noninvasive temporary cardiac pacing. J Electrophysiol 1:156, 1987.
5. Altamura G, Boocadamo R, Toscan S, et al.: Treatment of brady and tachyarrhythmias by means of transcutaneous pacing (Abstr). Cardiostimolazione 4:213, 1986.
6. Rosenthal M, Stamato N, Marchlinsky F, et al.: Noninvasive cardiac pacing for termination of sustained, uniform ventricular tachycardia. Am J Cardiol 58:561, 1986.
7. Prochaczek F, Galecka J, Becker A, et al.: Value of the external transdermal cardiac pacing in evoking and terminating of supraventricular atrioventricular nodal tachycardia (Abstr). PACE 10:731, 1987.
8. Luck JC, Davis D: Termination of sustained tachycardia by external noninvasive pacing. PACE 10:1125, 1987.
9. Falk RH, Ngai STA, Kumaki DJ, et al.: Cardiac activation during external cardiac pacing. PACE 10 (Part I):503, 1987.
10. Klein L, Miles W, Heger J, et al.: Transcutaneous pacing: Strength-interval curves and feasibility for programmed electrical stimulation. Circulation 76:IV-84, 1987.
11. Prochaczek F, Galecka J: The effect of the suppression time of the stimulating impulse artifact on the shape of QRS complex during transcutaneous pacing. PACE 13:2022, 1990.
12. Prochaczek F, Galecka J, Stanek K, et al.: New diagnostic prospects for

transesophageal pacing of the heart on the basis of an esophageal atrial electrogram received during stimulation. Stimucoeur 14:159, 1986.
13. Stryjer D, Friedensohn A, Sclesinger Z: Ventricular pacing as the preferable mode long-term pacing in patients with carotid sinus syncope of the cardioinhibitory type. PACE 9:205, 1986.
14. Stryjer D, Friedensohn A, Sclesinger Z: A new classification of cardioinhibitory response to carotid sinus stimulation. *In:* Cardiac Pacing and Electrophysiology. Belhasen B, Feldman S, Copperman Y (eds), R & L Creative Communications Ltd, 1987, p 287.
15. Baller B: Coronary vascular reserve under atrial and ventricular pacing. *In:* Cardiac Pacing, Electrophysiology, Tachyarrhythmias. Gomez F (ed), Editorial Grouz, 1985, p 535.

Chapter 15

A Multipurpose Self-Adhesive Patch Electrode Capable of External Pacing, Cardioversion/Defibrillation and 12-Lead Electrocardiogram

John R. Windle, MD, Arthur R. Easley Jr., MD, Robert S. Stratbucker, MD, PhD

From inception of Advanced Cardiac Life Support (ACLS) from in Lincoln, Nebraska two decades ago[1] to the present reality of squads of emergency medical technicians within minutes of nearly every village in the country with a fire barn, great strides have been made in the successful diagnosis and treatment of life-threatening medical conditions, especially lethal arrhythmias, outside the hospital. Several recent ideas born of space-age technology have made it possible to identify, monitor, and treat a great number of patients with potential cardiac catastrophes. One of these technical advances, the cellular telephone, permits transmission of both ECG rhythm strips and diagnostic 12-lead quality electrocardiograms to hospital-based monitoring physicians within seconds of a squad's arrival at the scene for an emergency. This communication breakthrough had led several authors to advocate both the diagnosis of acute myocardial infarctions and the initiation of thrombolytic therapy on patients in the field.[2,3]

From *Noninvasive Transcutaneous Cardiac Pacing* edited by Pierre Birkui, M.D., Jacques Trigano, M.D., and Paul Zoll, M.D., © 1993, Futura Publishing Company, Inc., Mount Kisco, NY.

To facilitate the expeditious handling of expectant cardiac conditions in the field, a new electrode system was designed and fabricated by Marquette Electronics, Inc. Milwaukee, Wisconsin (USA). This system is designed to allow even a minimally trained emergency medical technician to accomplish transthoracic pacing, cardioversion/defibrillation, and 1, 3, or 12-lead electrocardiographic recordings through a single, self-adhesive thoracic patch. Initially, this system was designed to facilitate the acquisition of emergency 12-lead electrocardiograms with negligible delay. Implicit in the system design was limiting electrode noise and artefact during adverse recording circumstances associated with ECG signal acquisition. In our experience, the routine acquisition of hospital quality 12-lead diagnostic electrocardiograms lead misplacement or electrode dislodgement has required the assimilation of very specialized training and experience by highly motivated ECG technicians. These problems are made much more difficult by the pandemonium invariably present during the performance of emergency cardiac care in the field. Additionally, any system developed must accurately reproduce ST segment changes to aid in the diagnosis of acute myocardial infarction and must be free of artefact and noise which could preclude the accurate interpretation of cardiac arrhythmias upon which life-saving therapeutic decisions depend. In addition, such a system should be able to deal adequately with the two most common arrhythmic complications of acute myocardial infarction: heart block[4,5] and ventricular tachycardia/fibrillation,[6-8] especially when thrombolytic therapy is contemplated.

Development of the Multipurpose Polymer-type Chest Electrode

The one technological advance in recent years which has clearly set the stage for a breakthrough in the multi-modality patient interfacing has been the development of the adhesive-conductive polymer films. These highly conformable materials have many desirable features not available with conventional metallic electrodes. One characteristic which is critically important when considering materials as candidates for use as a multifunctional interface is the ability of that material to limit the polarization effect; a practical example is the ability of such a film to pass a significant electrical current through the body without taking on the characteristics of a battery. These effects are often of such magnitude and duration as to render an interface incapable of serving as a low-level biopotential transducer immediately following pacing or defibrillation pulses. Another related feature is the apparent near absence in these films of a persistent memory to high current, defibrillator shock pulses such that subsequent shocks find an electrical milieu quite dissimilar to that of the first shock. Traditionally, the polymer-type electrodes are notorious for exhibiting this phenomenon. Additionally, the polymer-type electrodes demonstrate a refractoriness to the mechanical and electrical effects of hydration and dehydration. The association of a number of these desirable characteristics in one material makes polymer-based electrodes ideal for dealing with the diverse requirements of monitoring, pacing, and defibrillation.

As previously noted, 12-lead electrocardiography is beginning to emerge as an important adjunct to prehospital assessment of emergency cardiac care patients, especially as the use of thrombolytic therapy outside of the hospital continues to expand. However, the industry's major investment in present generation resuscitation devices and systems must not be underestimated. There is clearly a practical need to develop an electrode system compatible with today's defibrillator and pacer technology without forfeiting the important intrinsic capability of conductive polymers to serve both high and low level current functions in rapid time sequence and to improve on the immediate requirements for yet more discrete active electrode sites in the same electrode array. As a practical compromise, a 24-site, (4 rows high by 6 columns wide), array of discrete rectangular 6 cm^2 pledgets of conductive polymer each backed by an appropriate metallic interface tab was cast into a Z-shaped adhesive foam backing. This backing has the dimensions of the average human left hemithorax and overlies the standard precordial lead positions. The metallic backing tabs were each welded to a wire, the aggregate of which were terminated in a standard 25 pin, RS-232 computer interface connector (Figs. 1A and B).

12-Lead Electrocardiography

In clinical practice, the flexible electrode array can be quickly affixed to the patient by positioning the mid right-most electrode site over the V_1 position to the right of the sternum and simply wrapping the flexible Z-shaped assembly around to the left infra-axillary region

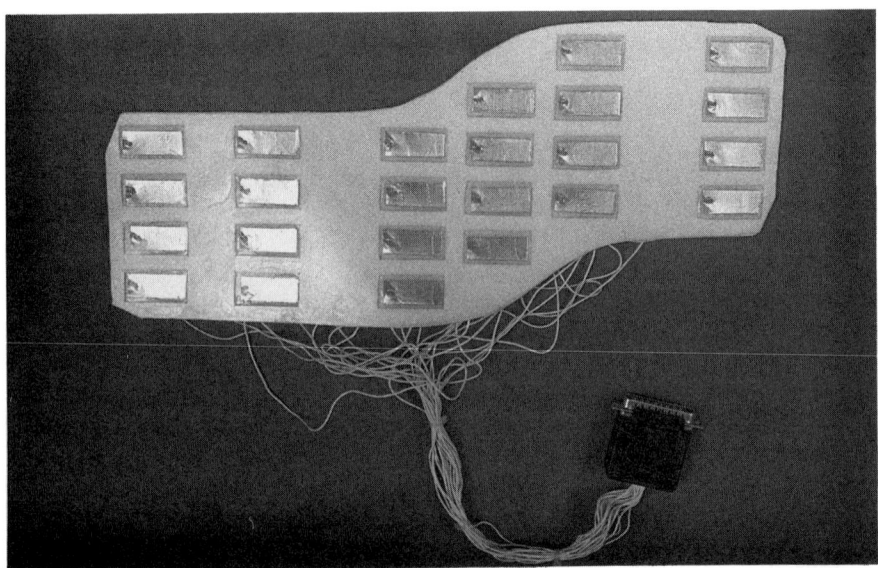

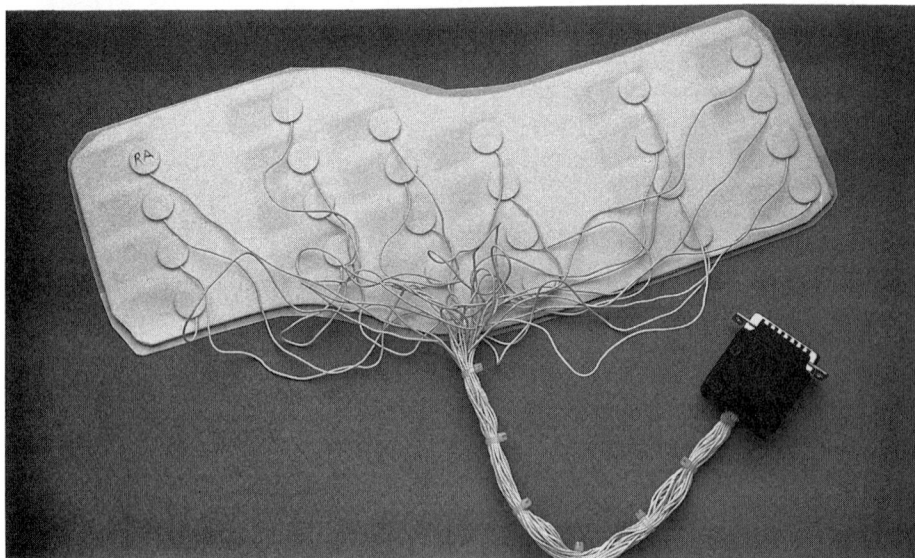

Figure 1. *The multipurpose, self-adhesive patch electrode. This Z-shaped (A, top), polymer-conductive electrode consists of 24 discrete pledgets (surface area 6 cm^2) arranged in 4 rows high by 6 columns across the precordium. The four corner electrodes serve as the limb leads. Each pledget (B, bottom) is connected to a terminal and standard 25 pin RS-232 computer connector.*

(Fig. 2). Standard 12-lead electrocardiograms taken without any mathematical correction for possible electrode misalignments were surprisingly free from distortion when compared to those of conventional electrode placement (Figs. 3, 4). In a preliminary evaluation in five normal volunteers, the measured heart rate, PR, QRS, and QT measurements were virtually identical (Table 1). Furthermore, precordial leads from the array mirrored the standard V_1-V_6 configuration in terms of amplitude, duration, ST deviation, and T wave configuration with medically insignificant error. The axis measurements were moderately inconsistent in patients two, three, and five. In the population tested, we noted no significant technical artefact or noise from the array. This finding may be of significant practical benefit when comparing standard 12-lead ECGs to those from this electrode array under field conditions where maintaining lead-electrode and elec-

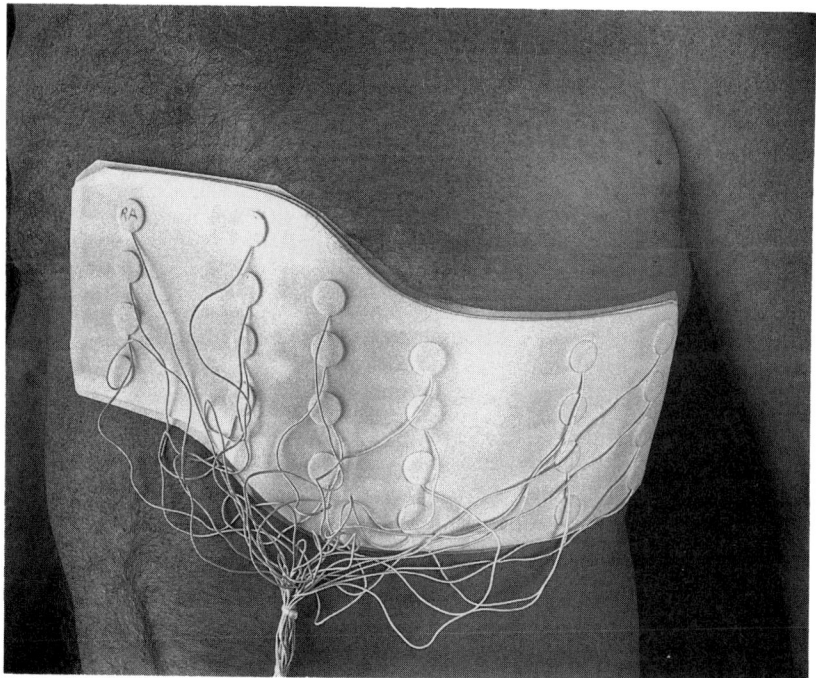

Figure 2. *The multipurpose, self-adhesive electrode. This figure demonstrates the positioning of the electrode over the left hemithorax.*

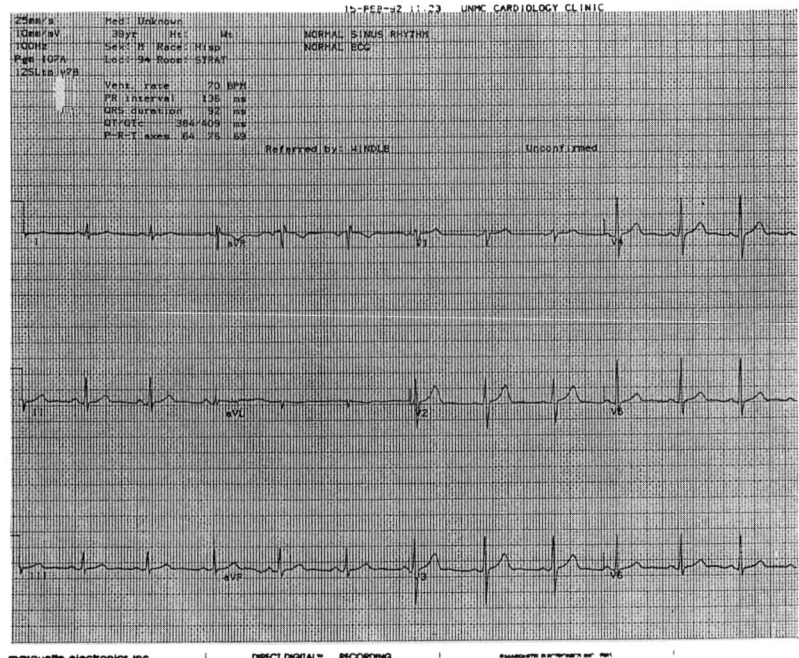

Figure 3: *Standard 12-lead ECG. The ECG demonstrates a normal electrocardiogram. The heart rate was 70 ppm, PR interval 136 msec; QRS 92 msec; QT 384 msec; and QTc 409 msec. Note the QRS axis of 76°.*

trode-skin contact for twelve independent lead wires simultaneously presents a very difficult task. The concordance between standard electrode positions and the multipurpose electrode's positions, and any corrective maneuvers required to reestablish the desired degree of exactness in both normals and abnormals is the subject of an extensive on-going investigation.

External Pacing

External pacing was performed in the same five non-sedated volunteers noted above. Transthoracic pacing was performed using a Marquette 1500 Pacer/Defibrillator. This device delivers a rectilinear, constant current pulse (5 msec rise) for 20 msec. Two arrays or clusters

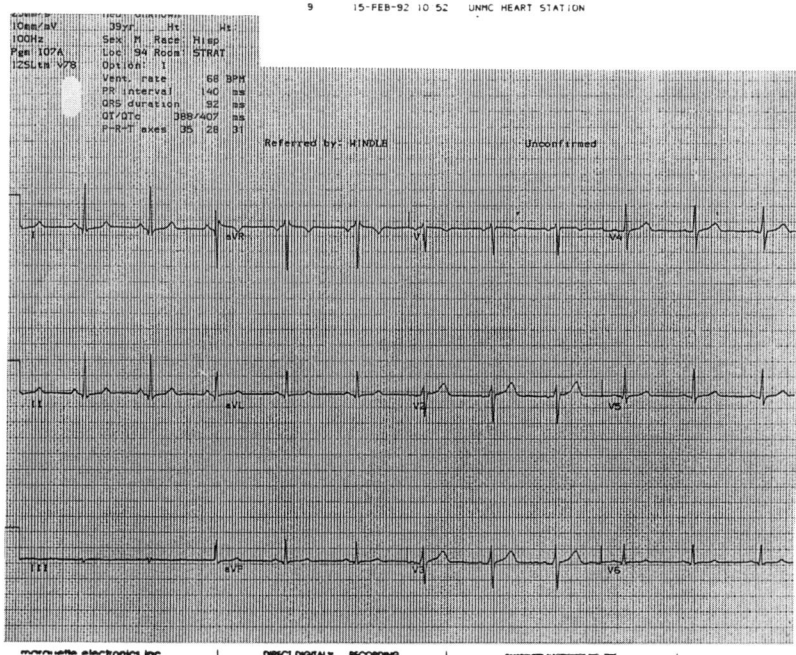

Figure 4: ECG obtained from multipurpose electrode. This ECG is from patient two and representative of tracings obtained with this electrode. Note the QRS axis is 28 degrees. The heart rate (68 ppm), PR interval (140 msec), QRS duration (92 msec), QT (388 msec), and QTc (407 msec) were not clinically different from the ECG shown in Figure 3. Additionally, the P waves and ST and T waves are easily seen.

containing six electrode sites each were wired in parallel, one array over the right border of the sternum, the second over the cardiac apex. Pacing was initiated at 30 mA and increased by 10 mA steps to a maximum of 120 mA. The apex was the negative electrode. Capture was achieved in three of the five volunteers (Table 1). In the remaining two volunteers, one was discontinued because of moderate to severe discomfort, and the second failed to capture at 120 mA. In these experiments, we were not able to test the more conventional anterior-posterior pacing position.

A visual analog pain scale with descriptors was used to quantify pain. Moderate to severe discomfort was noted by all volunteers. Their descriptors included burning, sharp, or stabbing pains. This

Table 1. Patient Results

Patient	HR (bpm)	PR Interval	QRS Duration	QT	Qtc	Axis (degree)	Capture Achieved	Current (mA)
#1								
ME	40	156	120	528	422	27	Yes	100
STD	38	168	112	548	429	19		
#2								
ME	68	140	92	388	407	28	Yes	100
STD	70	136	92	384	409	76		
#3								
ME	85	148	76	344	407	28	Yes	100
STD	87	148	80	340	408	−77		
#4								
ME	63	188	92	388	394	81	No	120
STD	65	180	92	384	396	84		
#5								
ME	65	136	100	380	392	23	No	80
STD	70	144	104	372	396	65		

ME = Multipurpose electrode ECG; STD = Standard 12-lead ECG. All values in milliseconds except as noted.

pain was not, however, significantly different from other electrode combinations, (Zoll NTP or Zoll pacer/defibrillator leads, and Marquette low impedance pads) tested in normal volunteers (unpublished data from our institution). Volunteers noted pectoral and occasional diaphragmatic pacing.

Defibrillation

The effectiveness for defibrillation of the multipurpose, self-adhesive patch was tested in six swine. The animals were sedated with ketamine (20 mg/kg) and xylazine (2 mg/kg) and ventilated on a respirator. The pigs were fibrillated using standard protocols of either transthoracic 60 Hz AC current in the range of one amp or low energy asynchronous defibrillator shocks. Following a 30 second delay, the animals were defibrillated with 200–360 J shocks using a Marquette 1500 pacer/defibrillator. All six animals were successfully defibrillated, generally by the first shock (Fig. 5). In addition to calculating the energy for each successfully defibrillation shock, the voltage and current wave forms were recorded and the per shock impedance was calculated for each animal using peak in-phase values of shock, voltage, and shock current. Of particular interest, the calculated transthoracic impedance for each active electrode cluster (where a cluster was six or more pledgets wired in parallel to form a single electrode) appeared to be constant as a function of the number of

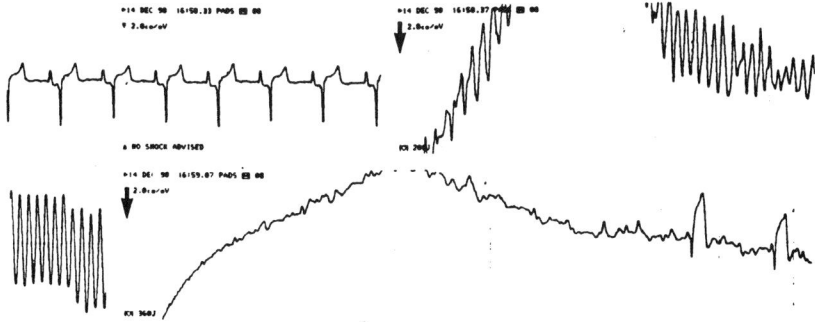

Figure 5: *Defibrillation of a swine. Following 30 sec of ventricular fibrillation (to trace showing reduction) one 360 J shock was applied through the multipurpose electrode to restore sinus rhythm.*

participating pledgets over a wide range. This value remained stable when we reduced the total effective area of each electrode cluster by 50 percent of its nominal value of 60 cm. At this time, the optimum number and optimum geometric configuration of these pledgets to reduce effective per shock defibrillation energy to a practical minimum is unknown.

Discussion

Studies of the multipurpose, self-adhesive patch suggest that a single, self-adhesive patch can successfully perform transthoracic pacing, cardioversion/defibrillation, and acquisition of 12-lead ECGs. We found that the 12-lead ECG produced by this configuration appeared to accurately mirror the standard ECG with sufficient fidelity to make accurate analysis of intervals and ST-T segments in normal volunteers. The variable axis shift may be explained by the shortened anteriorly positioned limb leads (the four corners of the pad). Further investigation will be necessary to validate its usefulness in ischemia and infarction, particularly with inferior wall changes. However, optimization of the patch configuration in conjunction with mathematical manipulation of the electrocardiogram recordings should allow for acceptably accurate diagnoses.

We found noninvasive pacing was successful in 60% of the volunteers. This appears to be consistent with some of the low impedance pacing systems evaluated by Heller et al.[9] They demonstrated 50% capture at a mean of 104 mA using the Lifepak 8 and similar results with other low-impedance pacing configurations. Previously, Zoll et al.[10] and others delineated three factors which they felt affected external pacing: (1) surface area, (2) pulse width, and (3) lead impedance. They found that larger surface areas captured at lower energies and reduced the pain of pacing (our surface area was 36 cm^2 vs the more common 60 cm^2). Additionally, Zoll et al.[11,12] and Geddes et al.[13] have found longer pulse widths and high impedance (around 500 ohms) patches increased capture at lower current levels with no increase in skeletal muscle activity. In general, Zoll et al. have achieved capture at less than 75 mA when using pulse widths of 40 msec and high impedance leads. However, defibrillation through these high impedance leads is not clinically useful.

A Multipurpose, Self-Adhesive Patch Electrode   189

We are currently investigating whether a larger surface area will be associated with greater reliability of capture and less discomfort. However as noted previously, neither larger surface area or high impedance leads affected capture rate or the level of discomfort in our experience.

As most studies[9-12] used anterior-posterior pad position, we were concerned that location may have affected the rate of capture. However, Falk and Ngai[14] found that anterior-posterior and posterior and parasternal-apex positions did not produce significant differences in capture when the apex was negative. As we had the apex electrode negative, the positioning of patches does not seem sufficient to explain our somewhat lower incidence of capture. Further study is necessary to clarify these results.

Our animal experiments with defibrillation seemed to adequately address utility and success of the low-impedance electrode to successfully defibrillate swine, even down to effective surface areas as low as 12 cm^2. It should be noted that we chose swine rather than canines because their hearts are more comparable to humans in size and orientation and are probably a truer measure of defibrillation efficacy than canine models. Approval to investigate the multipurpose electrode in humans is currently being sought.

Future Applications

The development of a multipurpose electrode may greatly facilitate our ability to perform further diagnostic and therapeutic intervention. Recently, several authors[15-19] described tachycardia termination with external pacing and even noninvasive programmed electrical stimulation.[20,21] Additionally, Murdock et al.[22] described pacing as an adjunct to CPR, and a device which can quickly switch from pacing to defibrillation may offer such potential. The 24 discrete leads available on the multipurpose electrode may further enhance our ability to detect myocardial ischemia or infarction via body surface mapping techniques and even allow high-resolution signal-averaged electrocardiograms to be obtained. Further, work with transthoracic impedance may offer additional information about the hemodynamics of transthoracic pacing[23,24] and the ephemeral status of the cardiac pump in a code situation.

Conclusion

As pointed out by Drs. Luck and Markel,[21] external pacing may indeed be in its renaissance. The pioneering work of Zoll[25] now seems to be able to be integrated with the technologies of digital transmission of electrocardiograms, automated detection, and treatment of ventricular fibrillation and advanced polymer technology to bring the patient a step closer to the physicians. While significant refinements and clinical evaluations are still necessary, our preliminary studies show that the multipurpose, self-adhesive patch electrode is capable of recording a high quality, 12-lead electrocardiogram while also retaining the capabilities of transthoracic pacing and defibrillation, although much further work needs to be done to enhance, refine, and validate its capabilities.

References

1. Carveth SW: Cardiac resuscitation at the Nebraska football stadium. Dis Chest 53:8, 1968.
2. Holmberg S, Hjalmarson A, Swedberg K, et al.: Very early thrombolytic therapy and suspected acute myocardial infarction. Am J Cardiol 65:401, 1990.
3. Atkins JM, Leshin SJ, Blomqvist G, et al.: Ventricular conduction blocks and sudden death in acute myocardial infarction: Potential, indications for pacing. N Engl J Med 288:284, 1973.
4. Arntz T, Stern R, Linderer T, et al.: Efficiency of a physician-directed emergency medical system for prehospital thrombolysis in acute myocardial infarction. Circulation 84:2269, 1991.
5. Iserli LT, Humphrey SB, Siner EJ: Prehospital bradyasystolic cardiac arrest. Ann Intern Med 88:741, 1978.
6. Cobb LA, Conn RD, Samson WE: Prehospital coronary care: The role of rapid response, mobile intensive coronary care system. Circulation 44 (Suppl II):45, 1971.
7. Lawrie DM, Higgins MR, Godman MG, et al.: Ventricular fibrillation complicating acute myocardial infarction. Lancet 2:523, 1968.
8. Lie KI, Liem KL, Durrer D: Management in hospital of ventricular fibrilation complicating acute myocardial infarction. Br Heart J (Suppl) 40:78, 1978.
9. Heller MB, Peterson J, Ilhahpamipaur K, et al.: A comparative study of five transcutaneous pacing devices in unanesthetized human volunteers. Pre-hosp Disaster Med 4:15, 1989.
10. Zoll PM, Zoll RH, Belgard AH: External noninvasive electric stimulation of the heart. Crit Care Med 9:393, 1981.

11. Zoll PM, Zoll RH, Falk RH, et al.: External noninvasive temporary cardiac pacing: Clinical trials. Circulation 71:937, 1985.
12. Falk RH, Zoll PM, Zoll RH: Safety and efficacy of noninvasive cardiac pacing. A preliminary report. N Engl J Med 309:1166, 1983.
13. Geddes LA, Babbs CF, Voorhees WD, et al.: Choice of the optimum pulse duration for precordial cardiac pacing: A theoretical study. PACE 8:862, 1985.
14. Falk RH, Ngai STA: External cardiac pacing: Influence of electrode placement on pacing threshold. Crit Care Med 14:931, 1986.
15. Beaudry PR, Rosengarten MD, Nadeau L: Termination of ventricular tachycardia with transcutaneous cardiac pacing. Can Med Assoc J 134:145, 1986.
16. Rosenthal M, Stamato N, Marchlinsky FE, et al.: Noninvasive cardiac pacing for termination of sustained, uniform ventricular tachycardia. Am J Cardiol 58:561, 1986.
17. Barold SS, Falkoff MD, Ong LS, et al.: Termination of ventricular tachycardia by transcutaneous cardiac pacing. Am Heart J 114:180, 1987.
18. Luck JC, Grubb BP, Artman SE, et al.: Termination of sustained ventricular tachycardia by external noninvasive pacing. Am J Cardiol 61:574, 1988.
19. Estes NAM III, Deering TF, Manolis AS, et al.: External cardiac programmed stimulation for noninvasive termination of sustained supraventricular and ventricular tachycardia. Am J Cardiol 63:177, 1989.
20. Klein LS, Miles WM, Heger JJ, et al.: Transcutaneous pacing: Patient tolerance, strength-interval relations and feasibility for programmed electrical stimulation. Am J Cardiol 62:1126, 1988.
21. Luck JC, Markel ML: Clinical applications of external pacing: A renaissance? PACE 14:1299, 1991.
22. Murdock DK, Moran JF, Speranza D, et al.: Augmentation of cardiac output by external cardiac pacing: Pacemaker-induced CPR. PACE 9:127, 1986.
23. Trigano JA, Remond JM, Mourot F, et al.: Left ventricular pressure measurement during noninvasive transcutaneous cardiac pacing. PACE 12:1717, 1989.
24. Feldman MD, Zoll PM, Aroesty JM, et al.: Hemodynamic response to noninvasive external cardiac pacing. Amer J Med 84:395, 1988.
25. Zoll PM: Resuscitation of the heart in ventricular standstill by external electrical stimulation. N Engl J Med 247:768, 1952.

Chapter 16

Knowledge Systems, Expert Systems, Medicine, and Noninvasive Transcutaneous Cardiac Pacing

Fernand Vandamme, PhD, Michel Verheyen, MA

Knowledge systems in general and expert systems in particular are becoming widely used. The first big breakthrough occurred in medicine in the early 1970s. However, much has been changed since. One becomes aware rather quickly that several requirements have to be fulfilled for this technology to be of real practical use. Most important is relevant and ad rem knowledge taking into account the specific situation and the specific type of intended user. This requires an enormous amount of study concerning manual and automatic knowledge extraction methodology as well as user-friendly man-machine interface. Another important lesson learned from the 1970s, rather painfully in some cases, was that the knowledge technology or artificial intelligence approach has to be integrated as much as possible in the preexisting information infrastructure. Knowledge systems as a stand-alone must be the exception rather than the rule. Integration can happen in several ways. The knowledge system or expert system can function as an intelligent front-end, as back-end, or just linked to a preexisting data bank, if only to avoid copying the data that already exists in a main database.

From *Noninvasive Transcutaneous Cardiac Pacing* edited by Pierre Birkui, M.D., Jacques Trigano, M.D., and Paul Zoll, M.D., © 1993, Futura Publishing Company, Inc., Mount Kisco, NY.

In this chapter, we present the main knowledge function to be realized with knowledge systems and will illustrate their application in medicine. Finally, we will discuss their potential use in external cardiac pacing.

Main Functions of Knowledge Systems

Knowledge systems differ from traditional software systems in several ways. In the first place it is a question of methodology and orientation in development: knowledge-(in the most narrow sense a structure of variables) oriented instead of data-oriented structuring. Secondly, more and more knowledge technology is being used and integrated in traditional software systems, this makes the differentiation even more and more subtle.

The main functions of knowledge systems are interpretation, prediction, diagnosis, and therapy. These correspond with the main knowledge function (Fig 1). All of these knowledge functions are relevant for the most different domains of activities in industry as well as in the service sector (Fig 2). An understanding of these functions will help us to see the relevance of knowledge systems in medicine in general and noninvasive transcutaneous cardiac pacing (NTCP) in particular.

Basic knowledge functions are interpretation, diagnosis, and therapy selection. Let us take as a neutral (outside medicine) example, the repair of a malfunctioning car. We can make several types of observations. These observations must be interpreted, and on the basis of this, a diagnosis must be made. This requires cognitive skills with an enormous quantity and quality of knowledge. In fact, one could argue that observation, interpretation, and diagnosis are all variants of experience and knowledge-driven classification and integration but on different levels (Fig 3).

Knowledge systems can be very relevant for training novices in observation and interpretation, to make diagnoses, and understand the several subtasks of the therapy selection and action.

The targets of criticism are different as are the strategy and tactics to realize these jobs. But it is true that in both tasks, the same domain knowledge is relevant. This has as a consequence that the development of a knowledge system for support of experts or novices is a relevant base for the development of an intelligent tutoring system in

Main Knowledge Functions
Interpretation
Diagnosis
Prediction / Selection / Decision — Therapy recommendation
Training
Planning/scheduling
Quality assurance/control
Exhibition/marketing

Figure 1.

the same domain. Nevertheless, a hasty identification between both is a mistake.

Another important function of knowledge is its exhibitive (individually formulated) or marketing (socially formulated) function. Indeed, knowledge also functions to exhibit the outstanding quality of its "carriers, actors." As a result, these actors, or the organizations they represent, become more attractive. Rather recently we have seen that expert systems have also been used with success here.

Planning and scheduling is also an important function of knowl-

196   NONINVASIVE TRANSCUTANEOUS CARDIAC PACING

Domain Applications	
Medicine	
INDUSTRY	Business Management
	Marketing
	Product selection/configuration
	Engineering Research
	Production Planning Scheduling
	Manufacturing Process Plant Operations
	Physical Distribution
	Quality Control
	Customer Service
Accounting	
Finances	
Service Sector	Banking
	Assurances
Utility Firms Water/electricity	
Consulting	
Law	
Transport	
Selection	
Administration	
Etc.	

Figure 2.

edge. In any form of complex skills and behavior, the coordination among the several actions, the products produced or used, and the several actors implied in the production process of service is crucial. Today more knowledge systems are developed for dynamic planning and for scheduling complex actions, in view of unexpected disturbances that may arise and for a minimalization of the disturbances as well as for an optimalization of resources, time, etc. . . . The knowledge-driven planning and scheduling system is indispensable. Planning involves creating a scheme or method for doing or achieving

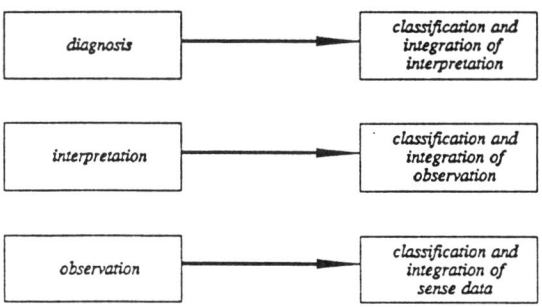

Figure 3.

a task. Scheduling concerns placing the planning in or on a schedule that allots time, dates, etc. . . .

Knowledge Systems–Application in Noninvasive Transcutaneous Cardiac Pacing

Intensive care, a relatively new concept in medicine, has developed in the last 20 years. It involves the continuous or very frequent monitoring of the "vital" functions of the patient, combined with the availability of several optional interventions that, when necessary, can be invoked on very short notice. Intensive care includes artificial maintenance of certain physiological functions (e.g., respiration, exogenous cardiac pacing, vasodilation) on a continuous or intermittent basis (e.g., hemodialysis). Any of these intensive care devices is a multiparameter-regulated system (i.e., its function is controlled by simultaneous feedback from several inputs and parameters).

The device to be discussed here is the noninvasive transcutaneous or external cardiac pacer, an assist device that supports the cardiologist in the therapy of a patient with symptomatic bradycardia or asystole. Rather than describing these devices, which are out of the scope of this chapter, we shall discuss their function from the standpoint of their needs for computer control and knowledge systems. The computer can be used for instruction and training in a variety of ways[1,2]: to manage instruction to test, to score, and to record student's progress, and then to assign new tasks with previous achievements.

Taking into account the earlier discussions on knowledge systems and medicine we can, among others, distinguish the following issues in the area of NTCP in which expert systems/knowledge can have a relevant contribution. Expert systems can improve the user-friendliness of information systems[3] and provide decision support for physicians.[4] With the combination of existing information systems and expert systems, many researchers[5,6] proposed the option that expert systems must be integrated with existing information systems to be successful and efficient.

*Knowledge systems for: transfer of relevant knowledge concerning cardiac pacing in general and NTCP in particular. The explosion of medical knowledge concerning cardiac pacing during recent years make it virtually impossible for attending clinicians to use all the information and knowledge available for making an optimal diagnosis. Even specialists in the field find it difficult to keep up with rapid developments in technology and clinical research. Knowledge systems can be used to store and disseminate different kinds of expertise concerning cardiac pacing (aspects of diagnosing, therapy, maintenance, etc. . .) in such a way that clinicians have fast and easy access to the relevant knowledge. From this viewpoint, knowledge systems fulfill the role of support device for information needs concerning cardiac pacing.

*Knowledge systems for: intelligent tutorial systems concerning training on several aspects of diagnosing, placing, control, consequences, social implications, etc. . . of NTCP.

In the early 1960s, researchers in artificial intelligence[7] had focused on problem solving in game playing, image recognition, speech understanding, and language understanding. During this time, some general problem-solving theories were formalized such as reducing a complex problem to a network of subgoals. However, it was discovered that most of the difficulties in achieving expert systems involved the need for computer programs capable of performing a task that normally requires the knowledge of an expert in the field. Four major programs were developed by 1975: PIP, CASNET, MYCIN, and INTERNIST.[8-10] Efforts to implement medical expert systems for routine clinical use inevitably require attention to the issue of human-computer interactions,[3,11-15] that have not traditionally been viewed as "mainstream" issues in artificial intelligence research.

The medical knowledge base can be an important tool for education in that it can form the basis for a number of intelligent computer-assisted instruction applications involving simulated patient encounters. For instance, the system can simulate a patient who suffers from cardiac malfunctions and the request for appropriate actions. The emulation of a real-life process on a machine permits compression of time, which in turn gives a student exposure to many situations. In knowledge-driven simulation, the student assumes the role of physician and the computer, the role of the patient. Knowledge-driven simulation falls into three basic categories: static, dynamic, and physiological models. In any of these formats, there is some facility for recording the student's performance for subsequent evaluation.

The **static simulation,** as the name implies, leaves the "patient's" condition unchanged throughout. A patient complaint and possibly some history are initially provided. The student interacts with the patient by choosing courses of actions from a menu displayed on the screen. History taking and examination can be requested from the menu, and results of information are returned as they become available.

In **dynamic simulation,** the "patient's" condition changes as a function of the student-physician's action. The changes generally are based on some decision tree and occur in discrete steps. Any action chosen from the alternatives presented will cause a transfer to another specified module somewhere in the tree. The computer reports any variance in the patient's condition along with some comment or criticisms. The next set of choices is then presented.

Many permutations are possible for a given case. The program can be designed to present cases in a random order, picking symptoms and situations that can be radically different from another case. In the domain of NTCP, dynamic simulations can introduce a real-time factor.

Physiological models combined with symbolic reasoning mechanisms are used to attempt to simulate a physiological system or disease process through underlying equations. If relationships can be experimentally established or developed, there is great potential for research and instruction. For instance, a student may manipulate variables of noninvasive cardiac pacing and then observe the reaction of the simulated patient system. The computer's ability to reason about complex situations can be combined with natural language dialogue to provide fast-paced experience using the mathematical model.

Knowledge systems for: support of cardiologist/quality assurance concerning the diagnosis and treatment of urgent cardiac malfunctions. One of the strengths of knowledge-based systems is that their reasoning mechanism is based on approaches that are systematic, complete, and consistent. This means that the system is capable of handling many parameters with no error and of coming up with a consistent response to any combination of inputs according to its knowledge base. This means it will better serve the patient in an emergency situation (which external cardiac pacing indeed is). A human may overlook a sign, forget to invoke a critical function, or act irrationally under stress, each of which leads to a catastrophic outcome in an emergency situation. In brief, in cases where a very rapid response is mandatory, such as in cardiac malfunctions and where the symptoms are not ambiguous, a knowledge system (that might include a critique function) would be acceptable to all parties concerned.

Knowledge systems for: supporting the cardiologist in the short-term and long-term management of patients who are at high risk for cardiac disease or who already have cardiac disease. For instance, information derived from clinical trials concerning cardiac pacing can be used in the diagnosis and assessment of the evolution of the patient state. It can also be used to help choose among alternative courses of action. Given the increased complexity of clinical-trial-derived data, there is a clear need to make use of knowledge systems to assist clinicians in the interpretation of clinical-trial data for diagnosis and patient management. Providing a result by clinical trial analysis is not an end in itself. In one way or another, analytical results need transformation into useful information within the clinical context in which the trials are performed. This transformation should yield interpretations appropriate to the context making it easier for the clinician to avoid misinterpretation of numerical data and providing "prompts" and even "opinions." An area of medicine where this need for enhanced interpretation of clinical trials is particularly acute is that concerned with the use of cardiac pacing in general and noninvasive cardiac pacing in particular.

The Use of Knowledge-driven Noninvasive Transcutaneous Pacing Devices

Effective regulation of all complex systems, whether living or man-made, depends on feedback and feed-forward. A feedback loop is formed by the sensing of key variables, calculation of appropriate system input in light of the desired setpoints and the current values of the variables, and eventually insertion of chosen inputs. Cardiac circulation in humans is a particularly effective form of feedback regulation, but when its limits are exceeded by cardiac malfunctions, it demands external support. To be useful, external feedback must follow the same three processes as internal feedback: sensing of key variables, determination of the level of appropriate intervention, and administration of the required input. Each element of this triad must be in place for any external regulatory pathway to be effective.

Next to the external feedback, we can make use of feed-forward systems. These systems are designed to maintain a desirable level of the therapeutic agent (for instance, the heart rate) in the appropriate organ system. When certain conditions (symptoms), which "predict" fatal malfunctions or inconveniences, are detected in a early phase, the system is able to provide suggestions to the cardiologist that will eliminate or minimalize the later onset of these disorders.

Through most of history, medicine lacked a repertoire of interventions of much benefit to the critically ill. Thanks to the advances of physiologists, pharmacologists, and bioengineers, such is not the case today. Cardiac malfunctions can be treated with drugs, noninvasive pacing, cardiac pacing, or cardioversion.

Today, the development of computers has facilitated the stimulation and control of cardiac functions with an unprecedented precision. We shall briefly outline an architecture in which knowledge systems can contribute to this effort. To realize this, we can set up an environment which is a knowledge-driven integration of three units, namely, an intelligent sensing unit, the knowledge-driven diagnosis and therapy unit, and the intelligent external pacing device.

As we have seen above, to be efficient, an external feedback and/or feed-forward loop must contain three elements: sensing of key variables, diagnosis (determination of the level of appropriate intervention), and therapy (administration of the required input). Knowledge systems can contribute to each of the elements in this feedback and/or feed-forward loop. At the level of sensing, signal filtering and signal processing, knowledge based systems can be used for the intelligent data compression of the electrical signal of the heart; at the level of diagnosis, the knowledge base can analyze the signals and assist the cardiologist in deriving a diagnosis; at the therapy level, it can suggest alternative setpoints for the external pacer. At the highest level, the knowledge system must contain a routine that is able to manage the communication between the three sublevels.

Sensing

In the context of this chapter, we interpret sensing as the use of external sensors to monitor these inputs. In relation with the electrocardiogram, these inputs are electrical signals originating in the heart.

Knowledge systems can be used at many levels within signal processing. At the lowest level, the system may be used simply to clean up or enhance the measure's signal and display it in a vivid and meaningful form. At the next level, the knowledge system may be implemented to extract from these signals predetermined features that preserve the medical significance while eliminating redundancy and irrelevant detail. These features may be of immediate interest to the cardiologist for further analysis and diagnosis. The intelligent removal of redundant and irrelevant information from a signal to create a simpler signal is called intelligent data filtering and compression.

In the case of NTCP, the knowledge system must be able to go beyond signal enhancement to some form of signal analysis. For purposes of the desired analysis, not all the details contained in the original (or enhanced) signal are relevant. The irrelevant detail should be eliminated as early in the processing cycle as possible, thus simplifying and speeding up the analysis procedure to follow.

Intelligent data filtering and compression is an important preliminary step in signal analysis, and it may dramatically reduce redundancy and unwanted detail and thus permit the subsequent analysis procedures to proceed more efficiently. Efficient implementation of this step in the cycle of data interpretation is often the difference between a system working efficiently with limited computing power and memory and delivery of its final display in a timely manner and one whose cost-benefit performance is unacceptable. This is also necessary for economical and efficient storage of the data.

Diagnosis

A knowledge system can be used to support human intelligence in the interpretation and analysis of ECGs and other data, which will be the basis for diagnosis and therapy. Using appropriate knowledge-based ECG pattern recognition programs, the function of the paced heart can be analyzed and, if necessary, the results applied to adjust the different operation parameters of the external pacer.

The features, obtained from data compression, may be abstract attributes of the signals that serve as input to classification and pattern analysis procedures. Here the system derives conclusions about the signal, based on the data itself and a knowledge base that puts the data into context.

Knowledge systems can extend beyond pattern recognition in two important respects: the knowledge base is assumed to be dynamic and highly diverse, and the operation of the system is in the form of an interactive dialogue with a human user. In relation to ECG analysis, for instance, we can expect the ECG to be input to the system and the medical user is expected to work with the system to define an interpretation. The system will interrogate the expert-user and occasionally in the presence of certain ambiguities, the system may display a hypothetical waveform and ask the expert-user certain questions to clarify the interpretation of the signal in question.

Therapy

The knowledge system can also support the cardiologist in the choice of therapy alternatives. In the case of noninvasive pacing, it means the setting of parameters for the external pacing device. The support might include an alarm to call for human attention to a noninvoked critical function, a warning to the cardiologist concerning an action that is not consistent with the internal knowledge of the system (critique function), the presentation of relevant information, the providing of advice concerning alternative actions that can be undertaken, the explanation and justification of decisions, etc. . . . This can be achieved by knowledge-based systems, given the appropriate knowledge representation and reasoning mechanism. Knowledge systems are able to represent the expertise of the cardiologist in a symbolic representation. By doing so, the restriction of numeric algorithm can be eliminated and the system used in a more dynamic and flexible way.

Conclusion

The benefits of the application of knowledge technology in medicine, in general, and in each specific subdomain are enormous. Still the efforts may not be underestimated concerning a careful knowledge extraction, and an efficient knowledge transfer to the user via an ad rem man-machine interface. But once this is done, there are direct and indirect benefits. The indirect benefit is achieved by the amelioration and optimalization of the structure of the target domain induced by knowledge technology. The direct benefits are obvious.

Acknowledgments: We wish to thank the following people who have contributed to the work described here: P. Birkui, W. Buylaert, C. Mortier, D. Vervenne.

References

1. Clancey WJ: Tutoring rules for guiding a case method dialogue. Intern J Man-Machine Studies 11: 1979.
2. Clancey WJ et al.: Neomycin: reconfiguring a rule-based expert system for application to teaching. Proceedings 7th IJCAI Vol 2, 1981.
3. Vandamme F: On intelligent Man-Machine interface. Bikit Library Bull 4:2, 1989.
4. Horowitz G, Jackson J, Bleich H: PaperChase: Computerized bibliographic retrieval to answer clinical questions. Methods Inf Med 22:183, 1983.
5. Van Bemmel J: A comprehensive model for medical information processing. Methods Inf Med 22:124, 1983.
6. Vandamme F, Vervenne D: Man-Machine interface for Expert Systems. Proceedings Expert Systems As An Aid for Planning and Fabrication in Production Engineering, Conference, 1986.
7. Vandamme F: A general description of expert systems. Communication and Cognition Artif Intell 2:1, 1985.
8. Buchanan BG et al. Rule-based Expert Systems: The MYCIN Experiments of the Stanford Heuristic Programming Project. Addison Wesley, Reading, MA, 1984
9. Chandrasekaran B, Mittal S: Conceptual representation of medical knowledge for diagnosis by computer: MDX and related systems. Adv Comput 22:217, 1983.
10. Buchanan B, Feigenbaum E: Dendral and Meta-Dendral: their applications dimension. Artif Intell 11:5, 1978.
11. Erdman H: The impact of an explanation capability for a computer consultation system. Methods Inf Med 24:181, 1985.
12. Vandamme F, Vervenne D, Haeffer A, et al.: Rules of thumb for developing expert systems. Communication and Cognition. Artif Intell 3:1, 1986.
13. Vervenne D. The MYCIN-History. BIKIT News Letter 2, 1986.
14. Mortier C, Verheyen M: Validated data bank and dissemination for prescribers: state-of-the-art of man-machine interfaces in medical applications. Aim Project A1020, Deliverable 16, 1989.
15. Shortliffe EH: The computer and medical decision making: good advice is not enough. IEEE Eng Med Biol 1:2, 1982.

Chapter 17

Noninvasive Transcutaneous Cardiac Pacing: Current Devices and Related Products

Jacques A. Trigano, MD, Pierre J. Birkui, MD

Recent technology[1-3] of noninvasive transcutaneous cardiac pacing (NTCP), increasing clinical use of external pacing, and development of prehospital cardiopulmonary resuscitation have led to an extended NTCP instrumentation, provided by numerous manufacturers.

Intended to be used in a prehospital setting, but also introduced in the emergency department, intensive care unit, and electrophysiology laboratory, this instrumentation covers a wide range of devices, configurations, and characteristics. Stand-alone units preserve simplicity and portability. Combination of pacing, defibrillation, and electrocardiographic monitoring results in a mobile unit designed for cardiac arrest resuscitation. Integration of this unit in a complete resuscitation system comprising other specific monitoring functions is also proposed.

In all devices, the main features encountered include large electrodes area, ventricular sensing, prolonged impulse duration and programmable current amplitude. In all circumstances, the clinical application depends on excellent electrocardiographic monitoring.

Energy programmability is used to reach and maintain stable pacing at the energy level just above the pacing threshold to enhance

From *Noninvasive Transcutaneous Cardiac Pacing* edited by Pierre Birkui, M.D., Jacques Trigano, M.D., and Paul Zoll, M.D., © 1993, Futura Publishing Company, Inc., Mount Kisco, NY.

clinical tolerance. Tolerable low threshold pacing is particularly needed for prolonged periods of permanent pacing in conscious patients. Electrode maintenance and battery life are also essential parameters for prolonged periods of pacing.

As a result, to ensure no delayed application and controlled efficacy, the general rules of noninvasive external pacing therapy must be perfectly known along with the specific characteristics of the system employed and related products. NTCP units are associated with important related products including the electrocardiographic monitor, the pacing and detection electrodes, the batteries and chargers.

Device Configurations

The configuration of a stand-alone unit is the original version, and has been provided by a number of manufacturers offering, in the prehospital setting, simplicity and portability (range: 2 to 5.7 kg). More recent models offer pace rate, heart rate, or alarm messages LCD display. All have incorporated a blanking circuitry filtering out the signal-distorting pacing stimulus to allow electrocardiographic monitoring with an associated monitor recorder.

These battery-powered units have a variable autonomy (range: 0.5 to 6 Hz), a function of the delivered energy and the battery life. The battery status is usually controlled by an LCD alarm message. The recharge time is variable, from 6 to 20 hours. A flying battery change during stimulation can be carried out in a few seconds in some devices. AC powered central charges up to four batteries. Twelve volt DC powered chargers can be used in vehicles. Some modular units are independent 9 V battery powered.

The pacer-defibrillator combination is intended to provide a complete cardiac arrest resuscitation system, with antibradycardia pacing, tachycardia termination, and defibrillation. In a few models, a single set of electrodes performs heart rate detection, pacing, and defibrillation. The system integrates a monitor recorder for clear electrocardiographic monitoring, and several other functions such as display and annotation of time, heart and pacer rate, energy level, and alarm messages. The combination with a defibrillator and a recorder may result in a built-in or integrated electrophysiological system and a relative portability allowing transport use.

Integration of the pacer unit in a complete monitoring system is a concept offering both configurations, each of the integrated modules, whether AC or battery-powered, being available as a stand-alone lightweight unit or interconnected with the other monitors. An electrocardiographic monitor and a defibrillator are the basic units, usually combined with a blood pressure, oxymeter or temperature monitor, or an endocardial pacing unit (Table 1).

From stand-alone inexpensive units to sophisticated multifunction systems, this instrumentation was recently changed. Many of the earlier stand-alone models are not yet available. Recent units introduce an integrated high-resolution monitor with pacing parameters and alarms display.

Pacing Parameters

According to the three-letter generic code of cardiac pacing, and considering only the ventricular chamber, the pacing mode is characterized as VOO or VVI pacing depending on whether ventricular sensing is presumed or not. The VVI, or synchronous pacing mode is available in all recent devices. Ventricular sensing is adjustable and asynchronous mode (VOO) is also available. A few rare units offer the VOO mode only. Using the ICHD code, identification of simultaneous atrial and ventricular pacing or four-chamber pacing is uncommon.[4]

Simultaneous atrial and ventricular pacing may be characterized as a DVI pacing mode with atrioventricular delay equal to zero. The five-position ICHD code may be convenient, however, to specify the device programmability and antitachyarrhythmia functions.[1]

The wave form is monophasic and usually rectangular, and in some instances trapezoidal or exponential. The pulse duration is usually 20 or 40 msec, and in a few devices programmable from 5 to 55 msec.

Considering the programmability range of all available devices, the current amplitude could be adjustable from 0 to 210 mA, according to the unit, with 5 to 10 mA steps, or continuously adjustable. The pacer rate is programmable from 30 to 180 ppm or continuously adjustable. High pacing rate and in some devices a frequency doubling function are available for overdrive pacing in tachycardia termination.

Specific units are designed to operate in conjunction with a

Table 1. Configuration

Manufacturer	Z M I			Physio Control				Marquette Responder	Odam	M R L	
MODEL	PD 1200	PD 1400	NTP 1000	Lifepak 8	Lifepak 9	Lifepak 10	Quick Pace	1500	2000 E	PAC-ETTE	360 SLX
Size											
Height	18	11	15	35	35.3	10.4	11	14.2	3.7	11.4	16.5
Width	32	33	30	40	29.7	40.6	22	25.4	13.5	27.8	35.6
Depth	42	31	38	29	31	37	34	46.7	10.5	27.3	27.3
Weight											
Kg	12	5.9	8.2	17	12.3	9	4.1	9.1	0.36	4	7.3
Lb	27	13	18	37	27	20	9	20	0.79	9	16
Combined Devices											
Scope	yes	yes	yes	yes	yes	yes	no	yes	yes	yes	yes
Recorder	yes	yes	yes	yes	yes	yes	no	yes	yes	yes	yes
Defibrillator	yes	yes	no	yes	yes	yes	no	yes	yes	yes	yes
Presentation											
Built-in	yes	yes	no	yes	yes	yes	–	yes	–	–	yes
Integrated							yes		yes	yes	
Stand-alone unit			yes						yes	yes	
Battery											
Operating time (hr)	2.5	3.5	3	1	1		2	1.3	4	4	2.5
Recharge time (hr)	2	2	16	20	24		16	2	4	16	5

Table 1 (cont'd)

	Osypka	Obream	EMG COR-PULS		*CRC PACE AID	*MEDAC	Cardio-tronics	*Bioelet-tronica			MDI*	*MDE
	500–500 D	NP 4 D	CES 9 AV	PULS NIP	53 B	300 M	ETP 180	Triad EP II	ST1	ST2	Trans-pace	Redi-pace
	10.3	10	12		7.6	12	10.16	5			9	
	25.7	21	36		22.4	23	21.6	15	–	–	20	–
	26.2	22	37		28.7	31	23	8			22	
	5.7	4	6.5	0.28	2.7	3	3	0.5	–	–	2	2.8
	12.5	8.8	14.3	0.6	6	7	6.5	1			4.40	6
	no	no	no	yes	no	yes	no	no	no	yes	no	
	no	no	no	yes	no	yes	no	no	no	no	no	–
	no	no	no	yes	no	no	no	no	no	no	no	
										yes		
	–	–	–	yes	–	–	–	yes				–
	yes	yes	yes	yes	yes		yes	yes	yes		yes	–
		10	10	2	6		6	2	–	–	–	–
	15											
	8	10	10		21	6	10	14				

* = not available.

programmable external stimulator for tachycardia induction and termination (Table 2).

Electrode Characteristics

Disposable, pregelled, adhesive pacing electrodes have expanded active surface area (range: 70 to 120 cm^2) and nonmetallic inner surface to transmit a uniform current density. An adult, as well as a pediatric size (range: 30 to 50 cm^2), are proposed in some instances for use with the same device. Electrodes are connected with integrated cables or connected with the electrode cable via clips or specific connectors.

Ventricular sensing and defibrillation usually require application of added specific electrodes, or a single set of low impedance electrodes ensures all the functions including heart rate detection, pacing, and "hands off" defibrillation (Table 3).

Table 2. Pacing Parameters

Manufacturer	ZMI			Physio Control				Marquette	Odam
Model	PD 1200	PD 1400	NTP 1000	Lifepak 8	Lifepak 9	Lifepak 10	Quick Pace	Responder 1500	2000 E
Pacing mode									
VOO	yes	yes	yes	yes	yes	no	yes	yes	yes
VVI	yes	yes	yes	yes	yes	yes	yes	yes	yes
Wave form	rect.	rect.	rect.	trapeze	expo.	expo.	trapeze	rect.	
Pulse duration (ms)	40	40	40	20	20	20	20	20	40
Current (mA)	0–140	0–140	0–140	0–200	0–200	0–200	0–200	30–200	0–150
Rate (ppm/min)	30–180	30–180	30–180	40–90	40–170	40–170	40–170	40–180	40–160
Refractory period (ms)	100	100	100	340	200–300	200–340	200–340	220–350	

Pacing Monitoring

Clinical application of NTCP is based on electrocardiographic capture confirmation. Using a specific circuitry, a clearly recognizable symbol of the stimulus artefact marks the time of stimulation and allows identification of ineffective or effective stimuli. Electrocardiographic monitoring is also used to adjust the current amplitude to just above the pacing threshold, ensuring both safety and clinical tolerance.

An associated event marker function is available in recent models to confirm pacing induced depolarization. Time, date, delivered energy, heart and pacer rate, ECG lead, and other status messages are also printed (Figs. 1–4).

Mechanical capture evaluation is based on pulse palpation and also on clinical confirmation of improved perfusion. Monitoring of femoral pulse and peripheral arterial blood pressure can be affected by muscle stimulation. Doppler flow monitoring and pulse oxymetry may be helpful.

Table 2 (cont'd)

MRL Pac-ette	Osypka 360 SLX	Osypka 500	Osypka 500 D	Obream NP 4 D	Obream 9 AV	EMG CES Cor-puls NIP	*CRC Pace Aid 53 B	*MEDAC 300 M	ALS-ETP 4 180	Cardiotronics Triad EP II	*Bioelectronica ST 1	MDI* ST pace 2	MDE* Trans-pace	MDE* Redi-pace
yes	yes	yes	yes	yes	yes	yes	yes	yes	yes	yes	yes	yes	yes	yes
yes	yes	no	yes	yes	yes	yes	yes	yes	yes	yes	no	yes	yes	no
rect.	rect.	rect.	rect.	rect.	rect.					rect.	rect.	rect. or sinu.		rect.
20	20	5–50	5–50	30–60	2–50	27–54	20	20		20	4	20–170	20–170	20	20
0–150	1–180	10–150	10–150	0–125	0.5–150 (overdrive 300)	0–150	10–150	0–150		0–150	75–200	10–210	10–210	50–210
30–250 250	30–180 250	40–150 150	150 (×2)* 150–300	30–300 200–600	30–200	50–150	50–160	30–180		30–180 300	40–100 300	30–180 300	30–180	60–300

* = not available; rect. = rectangle; expo. = exponential; sinu. = sinusoid.

Table 3. Electrode Characteristics

Manufacturer Model	PD 2200	ZMI NTP 2000	NTP 2100	Physio Control Quik Pace	Marquette	Odam	MRL	Obream ES 130
Form	front: circular back: rect-angular	front: circular back: rect-angular	front: circular back: rect-angular	circular		front: circular back: rect-angular	circular	circular
Area (cm^2)	front: 78 back: 111	front: 78 back: 111	front: 31.1 back: 53.4	78	67	front: 15.4 back: 19.5	78.5	50
Impedance (ohms)	<1	1 kohms	1 kohms	500 ohms			<500 ohms	200–300
Associated functions								
Detection	yes	yes	yes	no	yes	no	no	yes
Defibrillation	yes	no	no	no	yes	yes	no	no

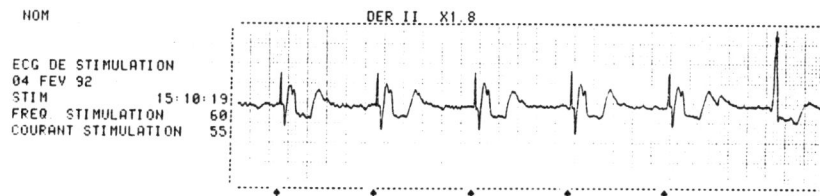

Figure 1. *Permanent demand pacing. Stable capture at 55 mA and rate 60 ppm. Arrows indicate pacing and a different symbol marks a detected spontaneous complex.*

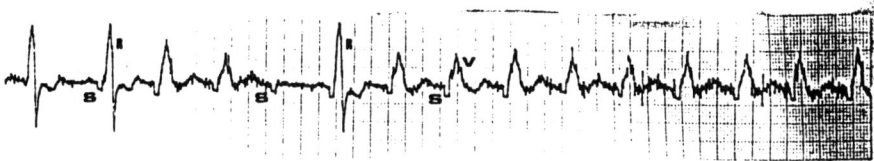

Figure 2. *Myopotential interference not preventing identification of the pacing artefact and the ventricular response. Permanent capture is preceded by a period with ineffective stimuli. The spontaneous complex R is intermittently preceded by an ineffective stimulus, resulting in a "pseudo fusion" aspect.*

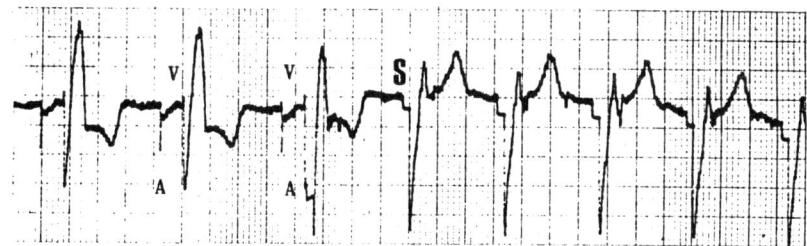

Figure 3. *Atrioventricular endocardial pacing (AV) in DDD mode at 70 ppm followed by external pacing at 90 ppm (S). The ventricular response is negative in the selected lead, with Sr aspect and large T wave.*

As compared to sinus rhythm or atrioventricular endocardial pacing, atrioventricular asynchrony induced by external pacing may have a negative incidence on systemic blood pressure, similar to that of endocardial right ventricular pacing. Hemodynamic changes related to atrioventricular asynchrony were shown in a personal study based on left ventricular pressure monitoring during NTCP.[5]

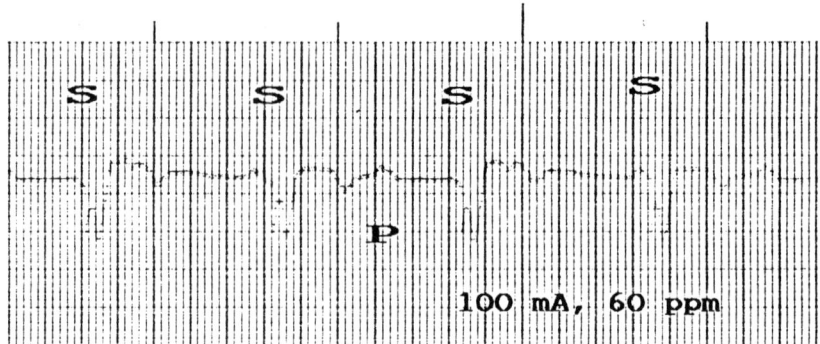

Figure 4. *Absence of atrial capture with persistent atrioventricular block evidenced by blocked atrial wave (P).*

An NTCP-induced pacemaker syndrome effect was suggested by the following hemodynamic findings: lack of a properly timed A wave in the diastolic left ventricular curve, cycle to cycle changes in systolic level, significant decrease in systolic index during NTCP as compared to sequential atrioventricular endocardial pacing (Figs. 5–7). However, a positive systolic effect may result from the skeletal muscle stimulation and from an adrenergic response.[6]

Clinical Application

The NTCP is an immediate and easy to use procedure for cardiac arrest or severe bradycardia in the prehospital setting. Its efficacy and tolerance depend, however, on the observation of a few general rules including the following steps:

1. Assessment of cardiac rhythm and baseline vital signs: Connect the patient to cardiac monitor and record rhythm strip. If using selective electrodes for detection, place the left leg electrode well below the level of pacing electrodes.
2. Pacing electrode application: Prepare clean and dry skin in the left anterior and left posterior positions. Shave excessive chest hair if necessary. Adjust electrode placement to conform to chest anatomy and musculature. Place electrode with negative polarity in anterior position. Use left anterior or V_2-V_3 position and left posterior position or epigastric area and V_6 position.

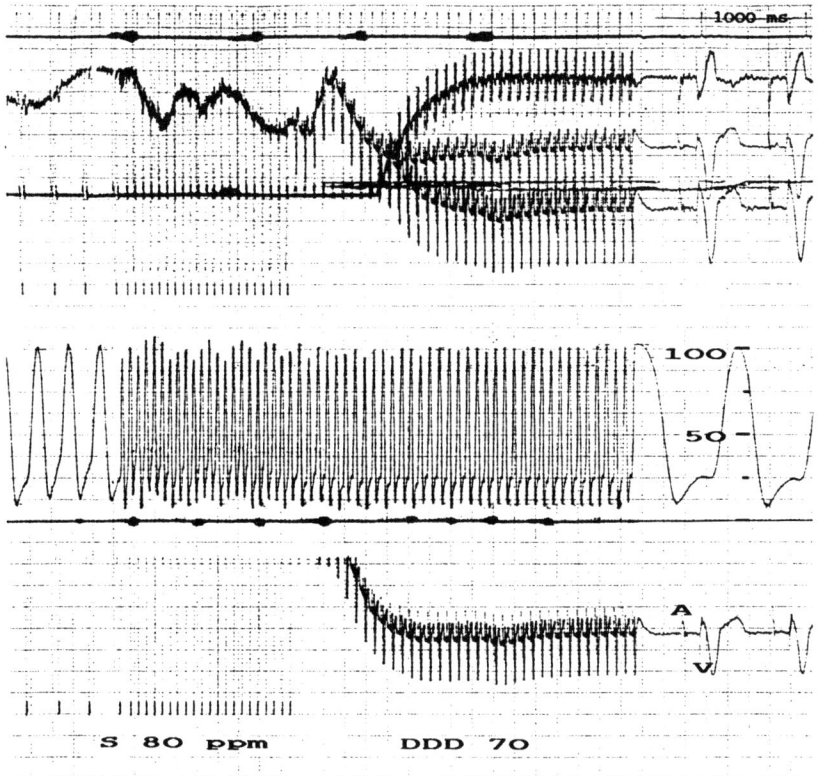

Figure 5: *Left ventricular pressure monitoring during external pacing. As compared to stability during endocardial atrioventricular DDD pacing, cycle to cycle changes of the left ventricular systolic pressure during external pacing is related to atrioventricular asynchrony causing variable timing of atrial systole before the ventricular systole.*

Check firm adherence of conductive surface of the pacing electrodes.
3. Pacing mode selection: If demand mode is selected, assure proper sensing of heart rate by adjusting the sensitivity control. With the pacer rate below the intrinsic rate and current amplitude at 0 mA, detection is confirmed by the QRS LED flash or the Marker Channel® of the recorder.
4. Pacing rate selection: Adjust the pacer rate above the intrinsic rate to measure pacing threshold, between 60 and 80 ppm.

216 NONINVASIVE TRANSCUTANEOUS CARDIAC PACING

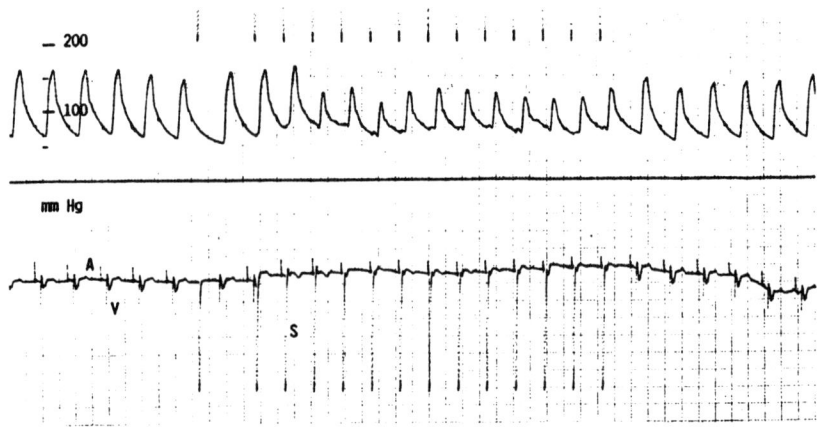

Figure 6. Femoral pressure monitoring. Marked negative systolic effect of external pacing as compared to preceding DDD pacing.

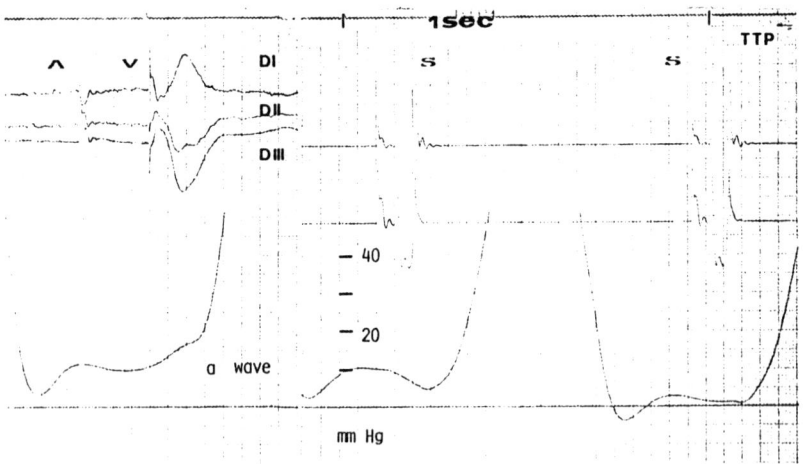

Figure 7. Left ventricular diastolic curve. Properly timed A wave during atrioventricular endocardial pacing and absence during external pacing.

5. Electrocardiographic capture: Increase current amplitude during ECG monitoring, and adjust amplitude to assume stable pacing just above threshold. Select ECG lead with clear pacing signal and ventricular response. In case of no electrical capture or high threshold with poor tolerance, evaluate electrode

repositioning, consider presumable etiology, myocardium viability, time delay of application, and previous pharmacological therapy.

Steps 3–5 require a specific knowledge of the device and of the manufacturer's specifications.

6. Tolerance: Observe chest wall muscle stimulation, and in conscious patients, clinical tolerance and comfort level. Consider sedative administration and patient reassurance.
7. Mechanical capture: Use femoral or carotid pulse palpation to monitor mechanical capture, showed also by improved level of consciousness and improved skin color and temperature. Differentiate between pulse and shock wave of muscle stimulation effect. In case of mechanical capture not following evidenced electrical capture, maintain basic life support and advanced cardiac life support to support circulation. Consider myocardial viability and metabolic status.
8. Maintenance: Consider the length of the battery life and its eventual replacement, the control electrodes and connections stability, and the quality of the electrocardiographic tracing. Monitor the correlation between tolerance and improved level of consciousness. Control spontaneous rhythm during a low rate pacing transient period. Consider low rate stand by pacing programming if appropriate to the clinical condition. Prepare transport and further therapy.

Consider the preparation of in-hospital transvenous pacing.
9. Tachycardia termination: Overdrive pacing is effective in terminating ventricular tachycardia. The limitations come from the poor tolerance of high rate pacing, rare incidence of atrial capture, and inability to select multiple ventricular stimulation sites. The use of an associated programmable external stimulation is to be considered.

Conclusion

NTCP is a fast and easy to use procedure for emergency cardiac pacing. Operation involves attaching the electrodes, adjusting the pacing parameters, and monitoring and confirmation of cardiac response. Successful application and tolerance are based on a few general clinical rules and on the perfect knowledge of the specifications related to each device.

Physicians, nurses, and paramedics should receive specific training regarding panel operations, electrodes, and batteries maintenance, and electrocardiography of cardiac pacing.

Instrumentation should include excellent electrocardiographic monitoring. Integrated defibrillation capability with multifunction electrodes enables a complete electrophysiological approach in cardiac arrest resuscitation including electrocardiography, antibradycardia pacing, tachycardia termination, and defibrillation.

Further developments should include enhanced electrode performance with device connections compatibility, and integrated mechanical capture monitoring.

References

1. Zoll PM: Noninvasive cardiac stimulation revisited. PACE 13:2014, 1990.
2. Luck JC, Markel ML: Clinical applications of external pacing. PACE 14:1299, 1991.
3. Kalk RH: Noninvasive external cardiac pacing. *In:* Cardiac Pacing and Electrophysiology. El Sherif, N, Samet, P (eds). WB Saunders, 1991, p. 675.
4. Parsonnet V, Furman S, Smyth NPD: A revised code for pacemaker identification. Five position pacemaker code (ICHD). PACE 4:400 1981.
5. Trigano JA, Birkui PJ, Degonde J: La stimulation cardiaque transcutanée thoracique. La Presse Médicale 3:124, 1992.
6. Murdock DK, Moran JF, Speranza D, et al.: Augmentation of cardiac output by external cardiac pacing: Pacemaker induced CPR. PACE 9:127, 1986.

Index

Activation, cardiac. *See* Cardiac activation
Advanced Life Support paramedic system, 75
Age, pacing threshold and, 20
Amiodarone, 122
Analysis of variance, 78
Anesthesia, 97
Angina, 171–172
Antero-posterior electrode position, 18, 22
Antiarrhythmics, 18, 134
Antitachycardia pacing, noninvasive transcutaneous, 143–144
Arrhythmia, 21, 143
Artefact, 93–96, 163
Artificial intelligence. *See* Knowledge systems
Asynchronous pacing, 52–53
Asynchronous ventricular mode, 21
Asystole, 54
    cardiac arrest and, 80, 82
    carotid sinus massage and, 169
    prehospital transcutaneous pacing in, 63, 75, 76–77
    results of, 80, 81
Atrial activation, retrograde, 164
Atrial capture, 6–8, 19
Atrial endocavitary recordings, 4–5
Atrial flutter, 109–113

Atrial stimulation, transesophageal, 170
Atrial switch repair, 97
Atrial tachycardia, 112, 113
Atrioventricular block, 25, 26, 164
Atrioventricular nodal reentrant tachycardia, 109, 135–139
Atrioventricular reciprocating tachycardia, 140
Atrioventricular reentrant tachycardia, 8–9, 109
Atropine, 76

Battery-powered unit, 206
Bipolar capsule electrode, 163
Bradyarrhythmias, 8
Bradycardia
    in child, 97
    indications for pacing in, 52
    pacing threshold and, 20–21, 22
    prehospital transcutaneous pacing in, 63–66, 75, 76–77
    results of, 80, 81
    resuscitation in, 51
    treatment of, 25, 26
Burst, endocardial, 114
Bypass tract, 9, 10

Capsule electrode, 163, 166
Capture, 15–16, 53
    cardiac arrest and, 53

Capture *(Continued)*
  electrocardiographic, 216–217
  failure of, 70–71
  mechanical, 217
  pacing threshold and, 93–94
  transcutaneous pacing devices and, 15–16
  12-lead electrocardiography and, 186
  ventricular tachycardia and, 142
Carbon dioxide elimination, 69
Cardiac activation, 3–11
Cardiac arrest, 49–60
  asystole and, 54
  cardiopulmonary resuscitation and, 56–57
  in child, 97
  contraindications to pacing in, 52
  cost of, 57
  defibrillation and, 55
  electrical capture and, 53
  failures of pacing in, 54, 55–56
  pediatric, 55
  prearrest indications in, 51–52
  prehospital pacing in, 54
  safety and efficacy in, 50–51
  survival and, 80–82
  technical considerations in, 56
Cardiac life support, advanced, 83–84
Cardiac output, 155
Cardiac pacing. *See* Pacing
Cardiac pressures and outputs in external cardiac pacing, 41–45
Cardiac rhythm assessment, 214
Cardiac stimulation, 14
  invasive programmed, 143
  noninvasive, 101–106
  noninvasive programmed, 132–133, 144
  pacing threshold and endovenous, 18
Cardioinhibitory type of hypertensive carotid sinus syndrome, 167–171
Cardiomyopathy, dilated, 108
Cardiopathy, 108
Cardiopulmonary bypass, 20
Cardiopulmonary resuscitation, 51, 82–83
  asynchronous pacing in, 53
  electrophysiology and, 101–103
  pacing during, 56–57
Cardiostimulator, 162–163
Cardioversion
  pacing in child and, 97
  tachycardias and, 112, 133–134
Carotid sinus hypersensitivity, 167–171
Catheterization in carotid sinus hypersensitivity, 169
CHB. *See* Heart block, complete
Chest circumference, 20, 93, 94
Chest electrode, multipurpose polymer-type, 180–181, 182
Chest pain, 171–172
Child, 91–98
  cardiac arrests in, 55
  electrodes and, 92–93
  indications for, 96–97
  pacing threshold and, 19, 93–96

Index   221

preparation of, 91–92
risks in, 96
technique in, 91–93
Chi-square test, 78
CK. *See* Creatine kinase
Concealed bypass tract, 9, 10
Conduction testing, ventriculo-atrial. *See* Ventriculo-atrial conduction testing
Congenital heart disease, 96
Contraction pattern, 152
Coronary insufficiency, 171
Coronary reserve estimation, 171–176
Coronary testing, 171–176
Cost of transcutaneous pacing, 57
Countershock, 101–102
Coupling interval, 127
Creatine kinase, 33–37
Current
    refractory period and, 127
    ventricular fibrillation and, 101–102
Cutaneous burn, 70, 96

Data filtering and compression, 202
Defibrillation
    multipurpose, self-adhesive patch electrode and, 187–188
    noninvasive, 101–106
    pacing after, 55
Defibrillator, 57
Demand pacing, permanent, 213
Demand ventricular mode, 21
Devices. *See* Instrumentation
Diagnosis
    knowledge-driven devices and, 202–203

knowledge systems and, 194, 195, 197
Diastolic curve, 216
Diazepam, 5
Dilated cardiomyopathy, 108
Discomfort
    in noninvasive transcutaneous pacing, 15–17
    in ventricular tachycardia, 142–143
Doppler assessment in echocardiography, 153–156
Dynamic simulation, 199

Echocardiography
    of left ventricular function, 149–157
    pacing threshold and, 20
Efficacy of pacing systems in cardiac arrest, 50–51
Electrical capture. *See* Capture
Electrical current
    refractory period and, 127
    ventricular fibrillation and, 101–102
Electrical shock, 70
Electrocardiographic capture, 216–217
Electrocardiography, 165
    of heart ischemia, 171
    multipurpose, self-adhesive patch electrode and, 181–184, 185, 186
    in tachycardia, 9, 10
    in ventricular tachycardia, 108–109
Electrode, 15–17
    application of, 214–215
    bipolar capsule, 163
    characteristics of, 210–212

Electrode *(Continued)*
  child and, 92–93
  electrical capture and, 53
  hemithorax and position of, 183
  impedance of, 24–25, 26
  localization of, 166
  multipurpose, self-adhesive patch. *See* Multipurpose, self-adhesive patch electrode
  in myocardial enzyme monitoring pacing, 35
  pacing threshold and position of, 18, 19–24
  polymer-type chest, 180–181, 182
  QRS complex and position of, 128
  ventricular activation and, 126
Electrode pad, 68
Electrophysiology, 99–145
  cardiac stimulation and, 101–106
  defibrillation and, 101–106
  fibrillation and, 101–106
  supraventricular tachycardias and. *See* Supraventricular tachycardia
  in tachycardia, 9, 10
  in tachycardia induction, 122–127
  ventricular tachycardias and *See* Ventricular tachycardia
Emergency management
  in cardiac arrest. *See* Cardiac arrest
  prehospital transcutaneous pacing and. *See* Prehospital transcutaneous pacing
Encainide, 134
Endocardial burst, 114
Endocavitary recording, 4–5, 7
Endocavitary stimulation, 3
Endovenous cardiac stimulation, 18
Enzyme monitoring pacing, myocardial. *See* Myocardial enzyme monitoring pacing
Epinephrine, 76
Equipment for prehospital pacing, 67–68, 78
Esophageal and esophagothoracal lead, 165
Exercise test, 171–176
Expert systems. *See* Knowledge systems
External pacing, 41–46, 184–187
External stimulator, 162–163

Feedback loop, 200–201
Feed-forward loop, 200–201
Femoral pressure monitoring, 216
Fibrillation, 101–106
Fisher's exact test, 78
Flecainide, 134
Flutter, atrial, 109–113
Four chamber stimulation, 3, 8

Heart block, complete
  pacing in child and, 97
  prehospital transcutaneous pacing in, 76–77
Heart catheterization in carotid sinus hypersensitivity, 169

Heart rate
  cardiac arrest and, 76
  Doppler assessment of, 155
  12-lead electrocardiography and, 186
Hemithorax, 183
Hemodynamics of external cardiac pacing, 41–46
Hypersensitivity, carotid sinus, 167–171
Hypertensive carotid sinus syndrome, 167–171
Hypothermia with bradycardia, 52

Impedance, electrode, 24–25, 26
Implanted pacemaker, 103, 104
  cardiac arrest and, 55–56
Impulse, QRS complex and, 163
Informed consent, 78–79
Instrumentation, 205–218
  clinical applications and, 214–217
  configurations of, 206–207, 208, 209
  electrode characteristics and, 210, 212
  maintenance of, 217
  pacing monitoring and, 211–214, 215, 216
  pacing parameters and, 207–210, 211
Interpretation, knowledge systems and, 194, 195, 197
Intubation of child, 91–92
Invasive cardiac pacing in cardiac arrest, 49–50

Invasive cardiac programmed stimulation for arrhythmia termination, 143
Ischemia, 108, 171

Knowledge systems, 193–204
  applications of, 197–203
  functions of, 194–197

Lactate dehydrogenase, 35–37
Latero-lateral electrode position, 22
Lead
  esophageal and esophagothoracal, 165
  monitoring, 68
Left ventricular function, evaluation of, 149–157
Left ventricular pressure monitoring, 215
LL. *See* Latero-lateral electrode position
Localization, capsule electrode, 166

Maintenance of instruments, 217
Mechanical capture, 217
Mechanical thumping machine, 104
Mobitz block, 164
Mode, selection of pacing, 215
Monitoring
  of femoral pressure, 216
  lead for, 68
  of left ventricular pressure, 215
  of pacing, 211–214, 215, 216
  systems for, 104–105
Motion-mode echocardiography, 149–152

Multipurpose, self-adhesive
  patch electrode, 179–191
    defibrillation and, 187–188
    development of, 180–181, 182
    12-lead electrocardiography and, 181–184, 185, 186
    external pacing and, 184–187
Muscle contraction, 67
Mustard operation, 97
Myocardial capture failure, 70–71
Myocardial enzyme monitoring pacing, 33–38
Myocardial infarction, 65–66, 108
Myocardium, 64
Myoglobin, 35–37
Myopotential interference, 213

New clinical applications, 160–178
  coronary reserve estimation and, 171–176
  hypertensive carotid sinus syndrome and, 167–171
  ventriculo-atrial conduction testing and, 160–167
Nodal reentrant tachycardia, atrioventricular, 109
  termination of, 135–139
Noninvasive transcutaneous antitachycardia pacing, 143–144
Noninvasive transcutaneous cardiac pacing
  cardiac activation by. *See* Cardiac activation
  echocardiographic evaluation of ventricular function during, 149–157
  efficacy of, 14–15
  history of, 13–14
  knowledge systems and. *See* Knowledge systems
  new clinical applications of. *See* New clinical applications
  pacing threshold and, 18–21
  for supraventricular tachycardia. *See* Supraventricular tachycardia
  tolerance and, 15–17
  for ventricular tachycardia. *See* Ventricular tachycardia
Noninvasive transcutaneous cardiac programmed stimulation, 132–133, 144
Noninvasive transcutaneous external stimulator, 162–163
NP-4D stimulator, 162–163
NTCP. *See* Noninvasive transcutaneous cardiac pacing

One- and two-tailed t-tests, 78
Oropharyngeal-epigastrium electrode position, 22

Pace Aid™, 4, 78
Pacemaker, implanted, 103, 104. *See* Implanted pacemaker
Pacemaker-defibrillator device, 67–68
Pacemaker pad, 68, 92–93
Pace rate in myocardial enzyme monitoring pacing, 35
Pacer-defibrillator combination unit, 206
Pacer protocol, 76–77
Pacing
  cardiac activation by. *See* Cardiac activation

Index 225

external, multipurpose, self-adhesive patch electrode and, 184–187
hemodynamics of external cardiac. *See* Hemodynamics of external cardiac pacing
mode for, 215
monitoring of, 211–214, 215, 216
myocardial enzyme monitoring. *See* Myocardial enzyme monitoring pacing
noninvasive transcutaneous antitachycardia, 143–144
noninvasive transcutaneous cardiac. *See* Noninvasive transcutaneous cardiac pacing
parameters for, 207–210, 211
permanent demand, 213
prehospital transcutaneous. *See* Prehospital transcutaneous pacing
rate of, 215
Pacing threshold, 18–21
child and, 19, 93–96
electrode positioning and, 21–24
in myocardial enzyme monitoring pacing, 35
Pacing window, 21–22
Pad, pacemaker, 68, 92–93
Pain
chest, 171–172
multipurpose, self-adhesive patch electrode and, 185–187
noninvasive transcutaneous pacing and, 15–17

prehospital transcutaneous pacing and, 67
retrosternal, 172–175
ventricular tachycardia and, 142–143
Pain threshold, 24
Paroxysmal supraventricular tachycardia, 120
Patch electrode, multipurpose, self-adhesive. *See* Multipurpose, self-adhesive patch electrode
Pericardial effusion, 70
Permanent demand pacing, 213
Permanently implanted pacemaker, 103, 104
Pneumothorax, tension, 70
Polymer-type chest electrode, multipurpose, 180–181, 182
Prearrest indications for pacing, 51–52
Prehospital transcutaneous pacing, 61–88
in cardiac arrest, 54
clinical use of, 68–70
complications of, 70–71
contraindications for, 66–67
discussion of, 84–86
equipment for, 67–68, 78
history of, 62–65
indications for, 65–66
informed consent and, 78–79
methods of, 76–77
results of, 79–84
statistical methods in, 78
systems in, 78
Programmed stimulation
invasive, 143
noninvasive, 132–133, 144
Propafenone, 134

Propranolol, 23
PSVT. *See* Paroxysmal supraventricular tachycardia
Pulse duration, 35
Pulseless idioventricular rhythm, 76–77
Pulse rate, 186

QRS complex, 93–96, 128, 186
Quality assurance, 199–200

Rate, pacing, 215
Reciprocating tachycardia, atrioventricular, 140
Reentrant tachycardia
  atrioventricular, 8–9, 109
  atrioventricular nodal, 109, 135–139
  supraventricular, 8, 110–114
Refractory periods, 124, 126, 127
Retrograde atria activation, 164
Retrosternal pain, 172–175
Rhythm strip of child, 93–96
Right upper-left lower latero-lateral electrode position, 22
RU/LL-LL. *See* Right upper-left lower latero-lateral electrode position

Safety, 21, 50–51
Scheduling, 195–197
Sedation, 91–92
Self-adhesive patch electrode, multipurpose. *See* Multipurpose, self-adhesive patch electrode
Senning operation, 97
Sensing, 202
Shock, 70, 101–102
Sick sinus syndrome, 97

Signal processing, 202
Simulation, 199
Sinus arrest, 168, 169
Sinus rhythm, 4–5
  atrioventricular nodal reentrant tachycardia and, 138
  carotid sinus massage and, 170
  echocardiography and, 151–153
  electrocardiogram and sphygmogram during, 165
  pacing threshold and, 20
Sinus syndrome of cardioinhibitory type, hypertensive carotid, 167–171
Skeletal muscle contraction, 67
Skin receptor stimulation, 67
Sphygmogram, 164, 165
Static simulation, 199
Statistical methods in prehospital transcutaneous pacing, 78
Stimulation
  cardiac. *See* Cardiac stimulation
  coronary reserve estimation and, 171–176
  endocavitary, 3
  invasive programmed, 143
  noninvasive programmed, 132–133, 144
  pacing threshold and endovenous cardiac, 18
  QRS complex and, 163
  transesophageal atrial, 170
Stokes-Adams disease, 119
  cardiac resuscitation in, 102–103

Index 227

Stroke volume, 155
ST segment, 174
Supraventricular tachycardia, 107–117
   discussion of, 112–115
   material and methods in, 107–109
   paroxysmal, 120
   reentrant, 8, 110–114
   results in, 109–111, 112
Supraventricular tachycardia, sustained, 131–140
   clinical data in, 134–135, 136, 137
   methods in, 132–134
   results in, 134–139, 140
Surgery, pacing in child and, 96–97
SVT. *See* Supraventricular tachycardia
Synchronous pacing, 52
Syncope, 119, 167–168

Tachycardia
   atrial, 112, 113
   atrioventricular nodal reentrant, 109, 135–139
   atrioventricular reciprocating, 140
   atrioventricular reentrant, 8–9, 109
   pacing threshold and, 20–21
   paroxysmal supraventricular, 120
   supraventricular reentrant, 8, 110–114
Tension pneumothorax, 70
Therapy
   knowledge-driven devices and, 203
   knowledge systems and, 194–197
Thoracotomy, 101
Thumping machine, mechanical, 104
Transcutaneous antitachycardia pacing, noninvasive, 143–144
Transcutaneous cardiac pacing, noninvasive. *See* Noninvasive transcutaneous cardiac pacing
Transcutaneous cardiac programmed stimulation, noninvasive, 132–133, 144
Transcutaneous external stimulator, noninvasive, 162–163
Transcutaneous pacing, prehospital. *See* Prehospital transcutaneous pacing
Transesophageal atrial stimulation, 170
Transposition of great arteries, 97
Transthoracic pacing, 49–50
Transvenous pacing, 49–50
Tutorial systems, 198–199
T waves, 93–96
12-lead electrocardiography, 181–184, 185, 186

Ventilation, 91–92
Ventricular arrhythmia, 21
Ventricular capture, 6, 142
Ventricular endocavitary recording, 4–5
Ventricular fibrillation, 101–106
Ventricular mode, 21
Ventricular pressure monitoring, 215
Ventricular tachycardia, 107–130
   clinical reports and trials in, 120–122, 123

Ventricular tachycardia
  (Continued)
  discussion of, 112–115
  induction of, 122–127
  material and methods in, 107–109
  pacing threshold and, 20–21
  results in, 109–111, 112
Ventricular tachycardia, sustained, 131–142
  clinical data in, 134–135, 136, 137
  methods in, 132–134
  results in, 139–142
Ventriculo-atrial conduction testing, 160–167
  discussion of, 164–167
  materials and methods in, 162–164
  results of, 164, 165
Verapamil, 23
VOO. *See* Asynchronous ventricular mode
VT. *See* Ventricular tachycardia
VVI. *See* Demand ventricular mode

Wolff-Parkinson-White syndrome, 134–135

Zoll NTCP, 15–16